D0162676

Marcel Bessis

Corpuscles

Atlas of Red Blood Cell Shapes

Springer-Verlag Berlin Heidelberg New York 1974

Marcel Bessis
Professor, School of Medicine, University of Paris
Director, Institut de Pathologie Cellulaire
Hôpital de Bicêtre, Paris, France

With 121 Figures

ISBN 3-540-06375-7 Springer-Verlag Berlin Heidelberg New York
ISBN 0-387-06375-7 Springer-Verlag New York Heidelberg Berlin

Composition: William Clowes & Sons Ltd, London
Reproduction and printing: Universitätsdruckerei Stürtz, Würzburg
Typeface: Gill, light
Paper: BBOT* Scheufelen, Oberlenningen
Dust cover and layout designed by J.Tesch, Heidelberg

Preface

The shape of an erythrocyte is determined by a delicate equilibrium of extrinsic and intrinsic forces. It may change during many pathological states as well as during a variety of experimental manipulations. Correct evaluation of the fine details of the red cell shape thus provides information of the greatest importance for the proper interpretation of the physiology and pathophysiology of many anemic states.

In examining red cells, the hematologist observes a drop of blood spread on a glass slide through the light microscope. This type of examination is likely to remain the routine technique of blood cytology for a long time to come. Still, we should not forget that blood smears are artifacts. The smearing flattens the cells completely, obliterating many of their characteristics and distorting others. It is therefore necessary to conduct a parallel observation of cells in the living state. The fundamental value of all such observations remains limited by the resolving power of the light microscope, which provides a maximum enlargement of one thousand times. To be sure, the transmission electron microscope can provide enlargements of one million times, but it lacks penetrating power, so that one has to section a cell into five hundred slices before observing it. The recent advent of the scanning electron microscope has changed the situation radically. As with the transmission electron microscope, the cells must be fixed, but they can be observed in their three dimensions and revolved before our very eyes, thus providing details of the surface and the shape of cells never before visualized.

The initial excitement over the new toy triggered a rush of publications, some of them overenthusiastic and uncritical. Upon examination, some of the new appearances of red cells were found to be at odds with those produced by more conventional methods. This inevitably raised the question of whether some of the new phenomena which have been reported might not perhaps represent artifacts, arising either during preparative handling of the cell or during fixation itself. Indeed, contrary to expectation, the long-lived red cells, which can be kept alive for several weeks outside the circulation and transfused successfully, are more difficult to fix without distortion than white cells and platelets, which were presumed to be more fragile because they are short-lived and less easily preserved for transfusion. Because of the importance of red blood cell shapes, it is certainly imperative that we know all the potential factors which result in artifacts.

Hematologists will not require a scanning electron microscope or even the much simpler phase microscope which permits one to study living cells in a fresh drop of blood. Having seen the results of studies with the new techniques, hematologists can now distinguish nuances in the appearance of red cells in routine smears which previously could not have been appreciated. Thus routine blood smears assume a new significance.

The Legends are numbered in accordance with the sequence of pictures in each chapter. The illustrations have been left unnumbered.

Table of Contents

On the Beauty of the Red Cell

On Nomenclature

On the Beauty of the Red Cell

The red blood cell is a living thing

All the illustrations in this album are pictures of red cells from human blood. Red cells are the simplest and best known of cells. Long believed to be nothing more than tiny sacs filled with hemoglobin which manage to remain in the bloodstream for one hundred and twenty days, these corpuscles have lately become the object of innumerable studies. Their chemical composition, their physical structure, the complex machinery which allows them to capture and transport oxygen, and the delicate mechanisms which govern the function of their membranes raise for the biologist many fundamental questions on the distinction between living and inanimate matter.

The very shape of red cells poses a problem. It results, as in all living things, from their code of inheritance and from the thousands of incidents encountered in the course of their brief existence. The experienced eye can recognize in the shape of a red cell either the subtle alteration of a gene transmitted from time immemorial or the scars of its daily life. The red cell which appears so simple is perhaps the first living thing which allows us to infer, by means of its outer form, its internal molecular arrangement. Its shape is a difficult language to interpret, but one we may be able to decipher eventually.

Some have made this pursuit their principal occupation.

Beauty is not easily defined

For those who are not microscopists, red blood cells are peculiar objects. Yet, glancing over their contours for the first time, one may experience a certain pleasure, a certain emotion, and may find in them a certain beauty. A theologian of the seventeenth century states that when one appraises beauty, one appraises order, proportion, and appropriateness. Perhaps some, as they view these pictures of red cells, will sense a law underlying the seeming haphazardness, a rhythm hidden behind the welter of accidents, a purpose within the variety of forms. Possibly they will perceive the element of time as well, for form depends on time—on the gradual and harmonious growth of its different parts in diverse directions. *Goethe* called architecture "music immobilized"; form is immobilized development.

Cells are living beings. Those who discern, even dimly, a law governing their forms at the same time also perceive their imperfections. "There is no excellent beauty that hath not some strangeness in the proportion," wrote *Lord Verulam*.

Imperfection is a part of beauty. What is perfect seems dull.

Beauty is not inherent in the object

"Take the statue you so much admire," said *Paul Valéry*, "move it to a land that is sufficiently different from your own, and it becomes nothing more than an insignificant piece of stone." The pleasure evoked by a work of art depends on the dialogue between the artist and the viewer, on the notions they both take for granted, on the conditions in which they have lived: the language which governs esthetic pleasure is not universal.

Nothing leads us to believe that nature intends to deliver a message to us. And yet, nature does use a language which is the same for all men, and which we may (or may not) yearn to understand. A rose, the trunk of a tree, or the song of a bird gives pleasure to both the untrained and the artist, a pleasure enhanced for those who make the study of nature their life's work. And so the beauty of red cells may move some, but how much more those who understand them! Countless notions accumulated throughout years of study: a beautiful picture, like the work of an artist, illuminates them in one instant.

Such immediacy is one of the graces of beauty.

Has the artist a foreknowledge of the laws of nature?

Is the resemblance between certain forms created by the artist and the shapes discovered under the microscope due purely to chance? The number of possible forms is not unlimited. The course of a river, the branches of a tree, the veins of a leaf, the ramifications of a coral reef, the dendrites of a cell are all built on the same model. Nature uses identical forms for different ends and on vastly different scales. The artist who expresses his feelings in shapes thus necessarily retraces the models of nature: certain sculptures by *Mirò*, who had never seen a red blood cell, look exactly like acanthocytes.

Or perhaps the artist creates these shapes because he has an instinctive awareness of the natural laws which govern forms. In other domains this instinct, the foreknowledge of the yet unseen, exists—or appears to exist. *Restif de la Bretonne* reports that at the age of three the sight of blood caused him to faint, well before the use of Reason could have given him the reason for it. *Mirò* does not know that his work is a marvelous illustration of red blood cells. Is that astonishing similarity inherent in the origin of art, or is it only an illusion that fascinates us?

One last remark: the pictures in this album have been chosen from thousands. Who is to say to what extent this choice has been influenced by what artists have taught us to regard as beautiful, by notions we have acquired, by earlier experiences, or by the preferences and aversions of those who took these pictures and arranged them on these pages. Are red blood cells beautiful or does this atlas merely display those we have found to be beautiful?

From the very uncertainty of the answer springs a special fascination.

Sir d'Arcy W. Thompson: On growth and form. Cambridge: University Press, 1959.

Paul Valéry: L'homme et la coquille. Paris: Gallimard, 162 (1937).

Paul Weiss: Beauty and the beast: life and the rule of order. The Scientific Monthly, 81, 286 (1955).

On Nomenclature

As the various shapes red cells can assume and their interrelationships begin to be understood, new names become desirable to codify the new knowledge.

The nomenclature used in this atlas has been the subject of lively discussion at a recent symposium. To paraphrase the arguments summarized by George Brecher:

Why new names? One may wonder if it is worthwhile to give a name to each odd form of the red blood cell. Acanthocytes can assume shapes reminiscent of a kangaroo, a "schmoo" of comic strip fame, or other fabled animals. The aim of classification could be defeated by the creation of special terms for each and every shape.

A new shape deserves a new name only when it is of sufficient frequency and constancy, or its origin of sufficient interest. Thus, as understanding widens, new cells arise or rather certain shapes can be separated from the welter of anonymous "poikilocytes." For example, not so long ago sickle cells were just "freakish red cells" and only very recently have acanthocytes and echinocytes been recognized as two shapes clearly distinguishable from other spiculed red cells.

Conservatism militates against new terms. Yet, having accepted the names created by our forbears for every red blood cell from erythroblast to reticulocyte, we ought to be willing to make additions as the need arises.

Why Greek? The principle of a universal nomenclature in an international language is favored by all because it is bound to aid communication. It may be argued that English is now the most widespread international scientific language. Still, non-English-speaking scientists (if this species exists) will find English no more evocative of red cell shapes than Greek, so that Greek remains the first choice in view of its long and successful tradition as the basis of international medical nomenclature.

The rationale of the proposed nomenclature: Classification of red cell shapes either by origin or by associated disease is impractical. For example, echinocytes and stomatocytes (or "cup cells") can be produced artifactually in a variety of ways, and they also occur in disease states. One basic name is desirable to designate identical shapes, whether artifactually or pathologically induced. At the present time, a classification by shape appears to be the only practical ordering principle.

The usefulness of compound names is also evident. For example, a whole sentence is required to describe in English an "acantho-cyte exposed to an agent which induces cup shapes in normal red cells." Stomato-acanthocyte conveys the same meaning in a single compound word. The prefix indicates the modification of the original form. Similarly, an echino-acanthocyte is an acanthocyte which has taken on the echinocytic form, and a drepano-echinocyte is an echinocyte which has sickled.

The compound nomenclature is also flexible. Should chemical distinctions between identical forms become possible, new names can be added.

Keys for the Nomenclature of Normal Red Cells

name	from the Greek word meaning:	definition
DISCOCYTE	*disc*	biconcave, normal, circulating form
Echinocytic transformation:		
ECHINOCYTES (I, II, III)	*sea urchin*	erythrocyte with spicules
SPHERO-ECHINOCYTES (I, II)		spherical erythrocytes with small spicules
Stomatocytic transformation:		
STOMATOCYTES (I, II, III)	*mouth*	cup-shaped erythrocyte
SPHERO-STOMATOCYTES (I, II)		small hilum or irregularity at the site of the invagination

Key for the Nomenclature of Pathological Red Cells

name	from the Greek word meaning:	Frequent in:
ACANTHOCYTE	*spike*	a-betalipoproteinemia and acquired hepatic syndromes
CODOCYTE (target cell = codocyte flattened on a smear)	*bell*	thalassemia
DACRYOCYTE	*tear drop*	thalassemia, hemolytic anemias
DREPANOCYTE	*sickle*	sickle cell anemia
ELLIPTOCYTE	*oval*	congenital elliptocytosis
KERATOCYTE	*horn*	hemolytic anemias, vascular surgery
KNIZOCYTE	*pinch*	hemolytic anemias, hereditary spherocytosis
LEPTOCYTE	*thin*	hypochromic anemias
MEGALOCYTE	*giant*	megaloblastic anemias
SCHIZOCYTE	*cut*	microangiopathic anemia, vascular surgery
SPHEROCYTE	*sphere*	hereditary spherocytosis, burns, some hemolytic anemias
SPHERO-STOMATOCYTE	*sphere—mouth*	hereditary spherocytosis and stomatocytosis
TOROCYTE	*torus*	generally artifactual

Some Figures Concerning the Human Red Cell

	in health	in disease
diameter (microns)	7.4 to 8.2	2 to 11
average thickness (microns)	1.5 to 1.8	0.5 to 5
surface area (square microns)	130 to 150	10 to 300
volume (cubic microns)	85 to 95	40 to 200
weight (picograms)	90 to 100	10 to 200
number per cubic millimeter of blood	4,400,000 to 5,400,000	500,000 to 9,000,000
total number (135 lb. man)	25,000 billion	2,500 to 50,000 billion
Life span (days)	110 to 130	0 to 130
Birth and death[1] (135-lb. man) per second	2,500,000	17,500,000
per day	200 billion	0 to 1400 billion
per average human lifetime	5 million billion (approx. 500 kilograms or 950 lbs.)	

[1] In the normal organism, red cells continuously wear out and die—having lived their normal life span—and are replaced by an equal number of newly formed cells.

Chapter 1

Red Cell Birth

Red Cell Birth

The red blood cell is derived from a nucleated cell of the bone marrow called an Erythroblast. On the third or fourth day of its development, when the erythroblast is nearly saturated with hemoglobin, it begins to have very peculiar spasms. It thrusts out and retracts numerous pseudopodia, one of them containing the nucleus, which, after a few convulsions, is expelled.

The inert nucleus is immediately engulfed by a nearby phagocyte.

The cell, after it has expelled its nucleus, is called a Reticulocyte. This young red cell is released into the blood stream, where its characteristic movements continue for one or two days, after which it becomes an adult red blood cell, an Erythrocyte.

In a normal human adult, 2,500,000 red cells are formed in this way each second.

Fig. 1. Erythroblast expelling its nucleus. The nucleus has just detached itself from the bulk of the cell which can be seen in the background with its characteristic wrinkles.

Fig. 2. Reticulocyte left after the nuclear expulsion. The appearance of this cell results from its characteristic movements, the mechanism of which is not yet known.

Figs. 3, 4, and 5. Reticulocytes. Microcinematography has shown that this aspect was due to sudden cytoplasmic expansions followed by slow retractions.

Figs. 6, 7, and 8. Echinocytic forms of reticulocytes. When they are placed in an echinogenic medium (see Chapter III) their surface bristles with spicules. These cells are very much alive, as shown by the persistence of cellular movements.

Fig. 9. Reticulocyte and mature erythrocyte. The contorted aspect of the reticulocyte contrasts with the smoothness of the erythrocyte disc.

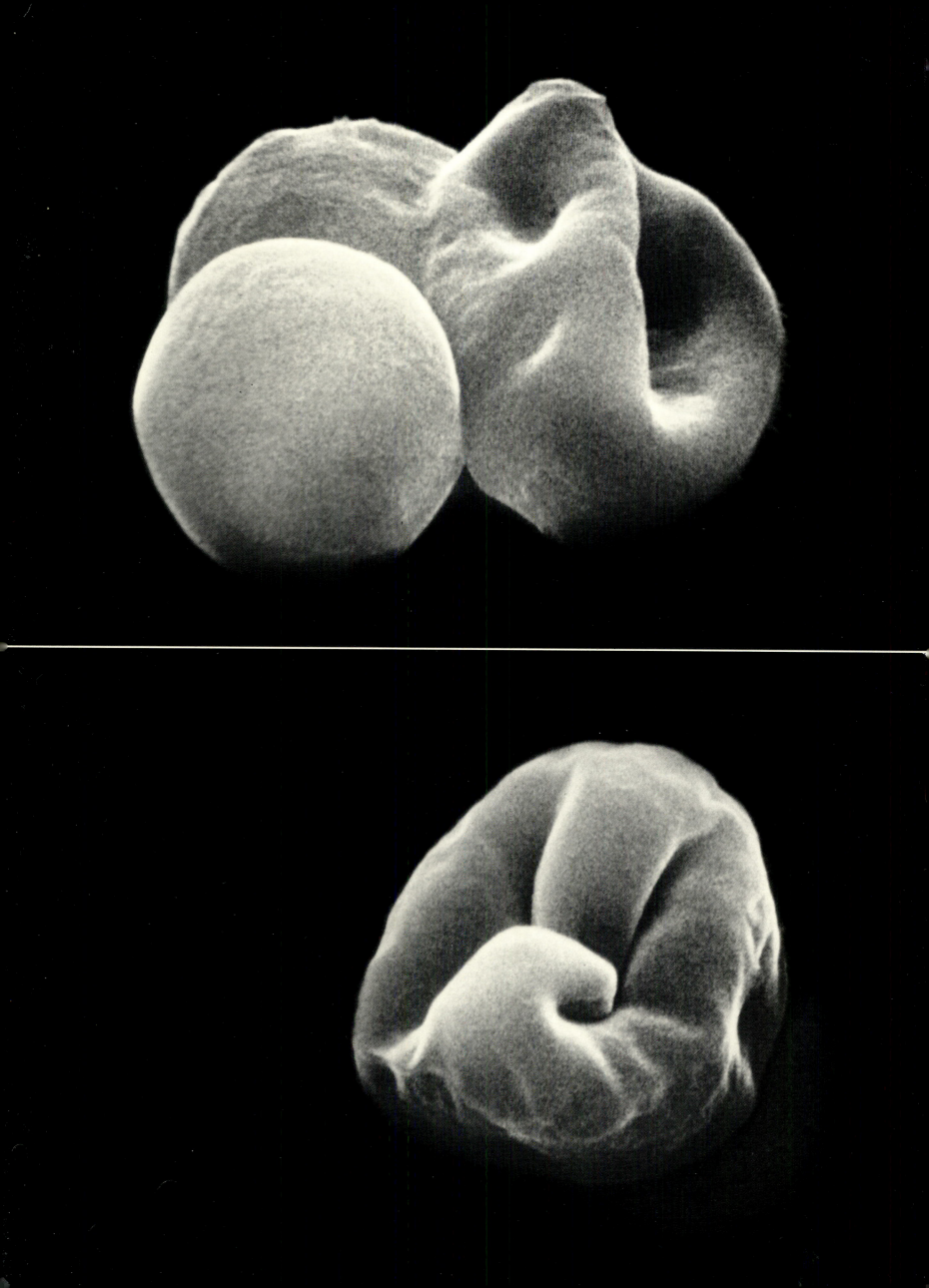

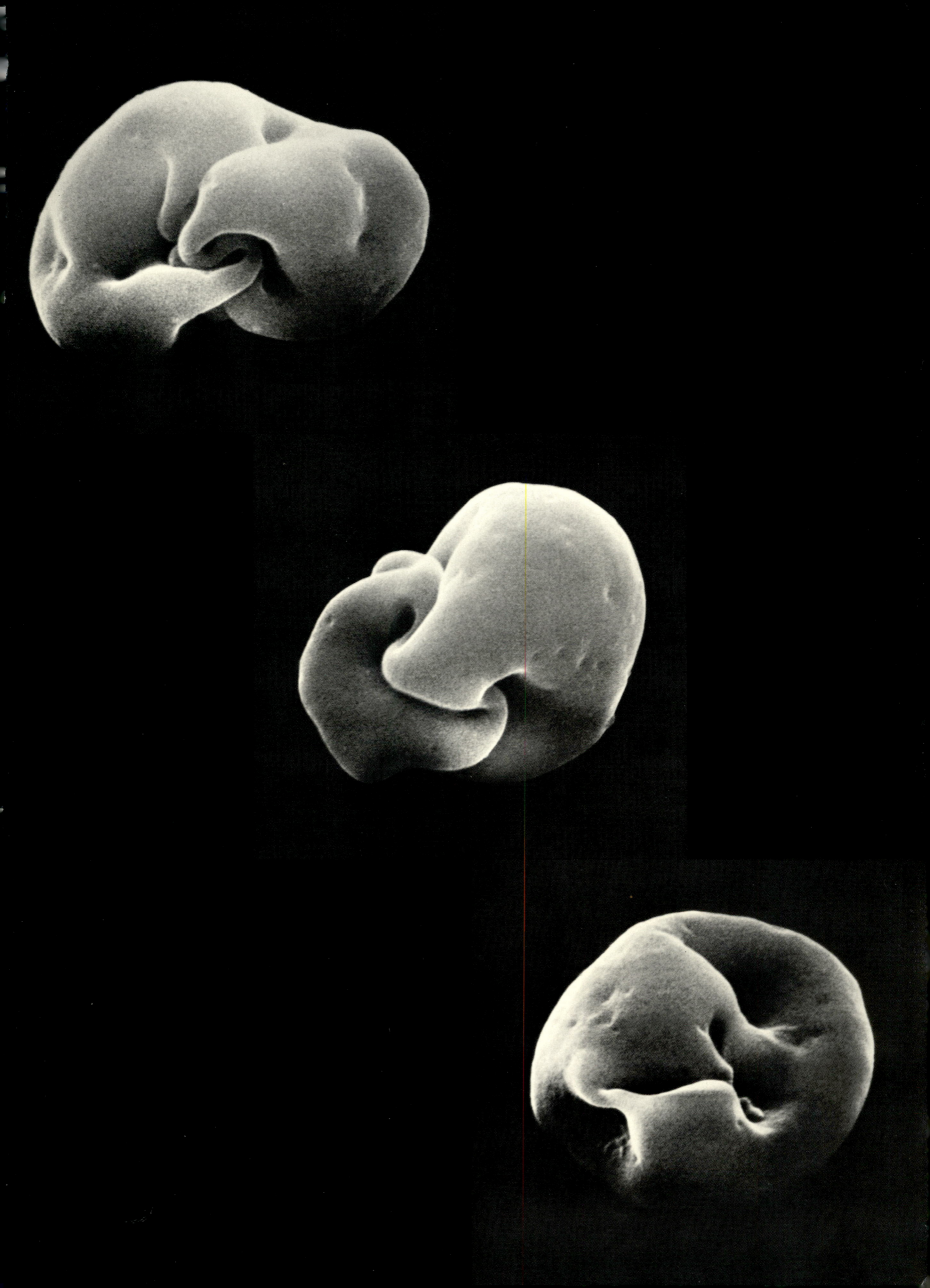

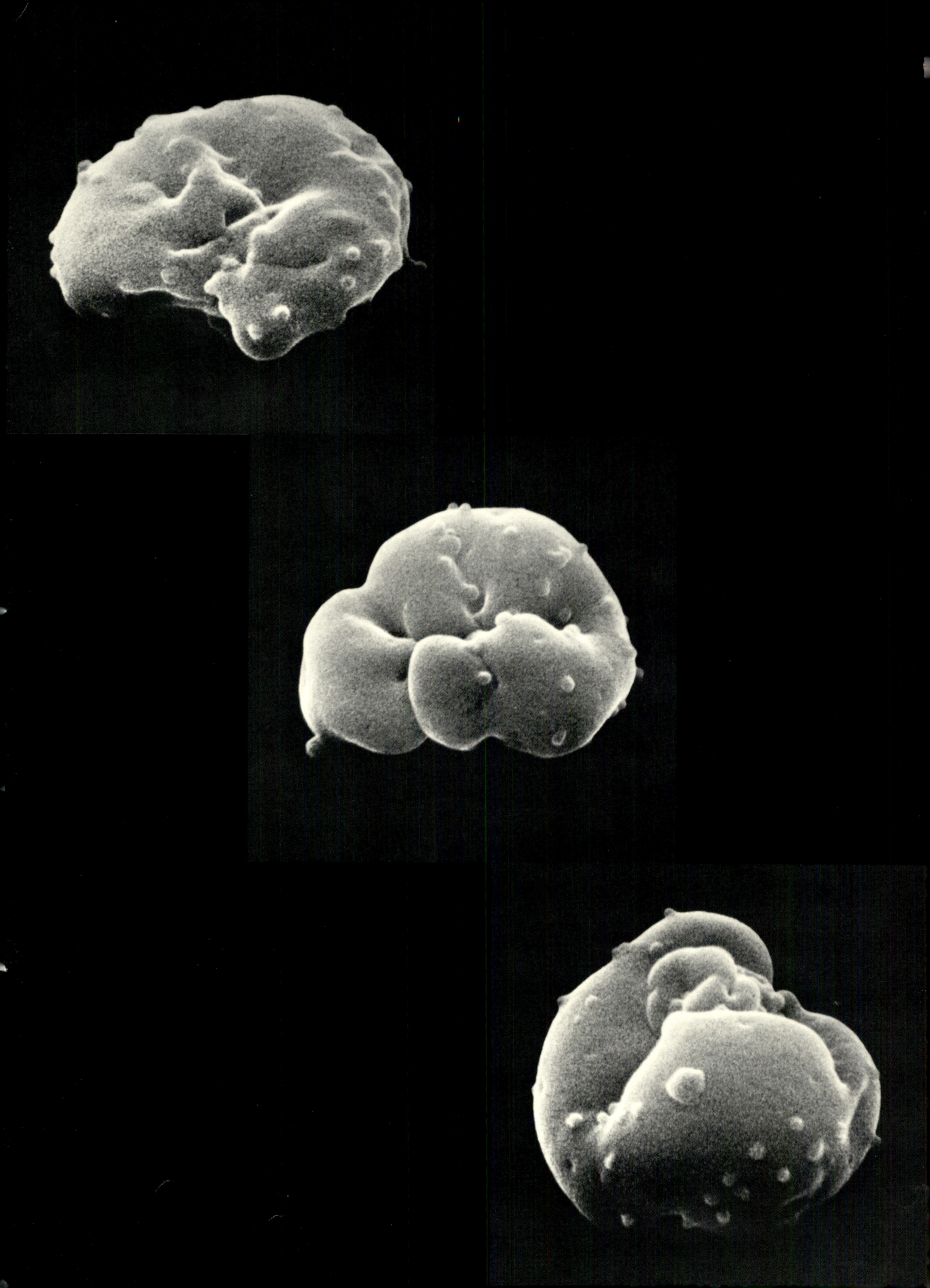

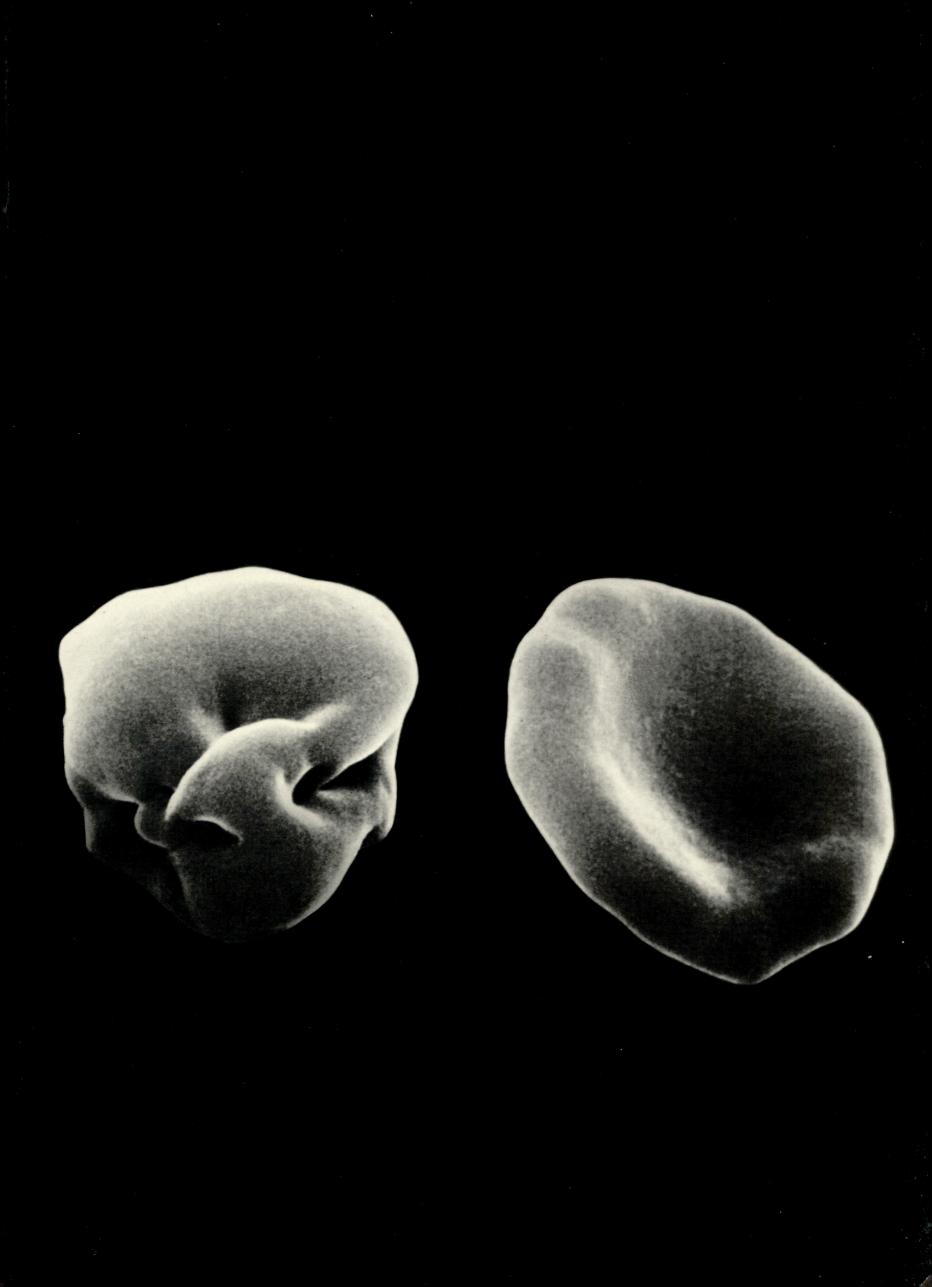

Chapter II

Discocytes

Discocytes

Normal human red blood cells have the shape of biconcave discs. Their dimensions are remarkably constant in a healthy person.

Discocytes are very deformable and also very elastic. In large blood vessels, red cells move in clusters, but in small capillaries with a diameter of 3 to 5 microns, they have to pass one by one. High-speed cinematographic studies have shown that during normal flow these red cells assume elongated parachute-like shapes, with the concavity oriented in the direction of the current. They resume their former shape as soon as they reach larger vessels.

The deformability of discocytes assures their passage through capillaries. Deformability varies with the metabolic state of red cells and may be decreased in disease. When red cells reach a certain degree of rigidity, they can no longer clear the finer capillaries of the lung, bone marrow, and spleen. Here they are trapped and finally hemolyzed.

Fig. 1. Normal red cells. They are biconcave discs.

Fig. 2. Discocytes on a blood smear.

Fig. 3. Cluster of red cells. Mutual pressures induce some deformations. One of the cells is an Echinocyte I (see next chapter).

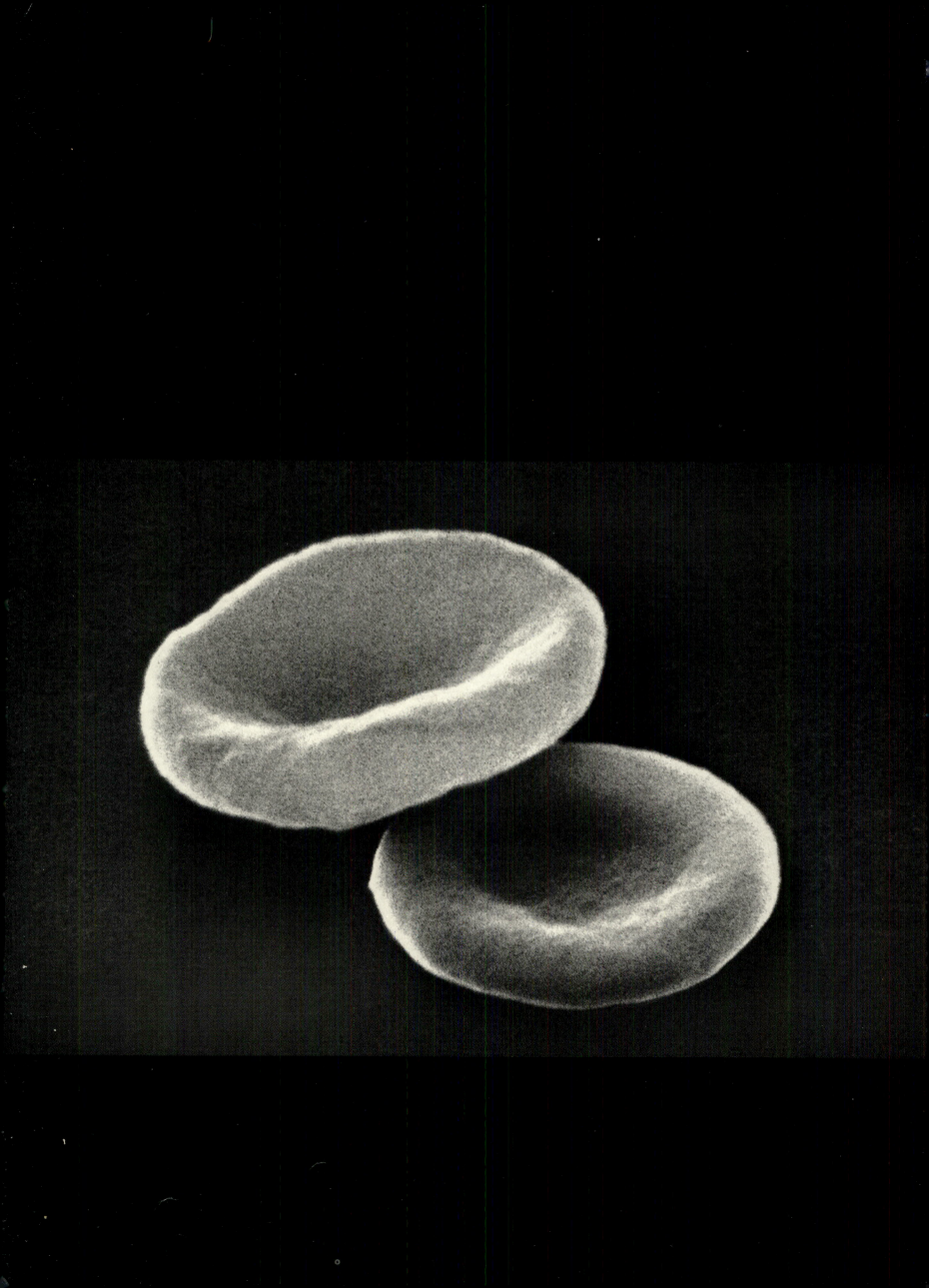

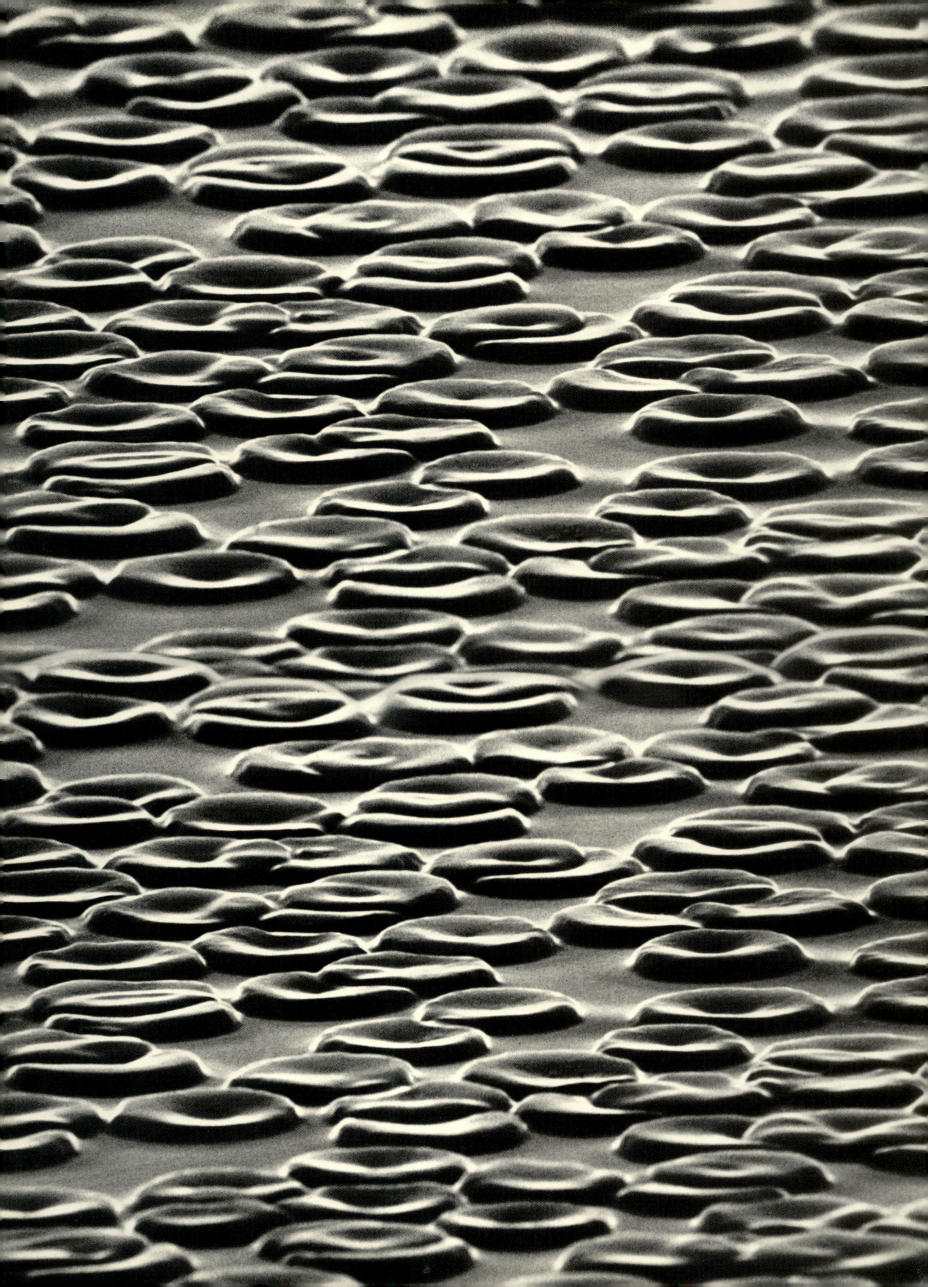

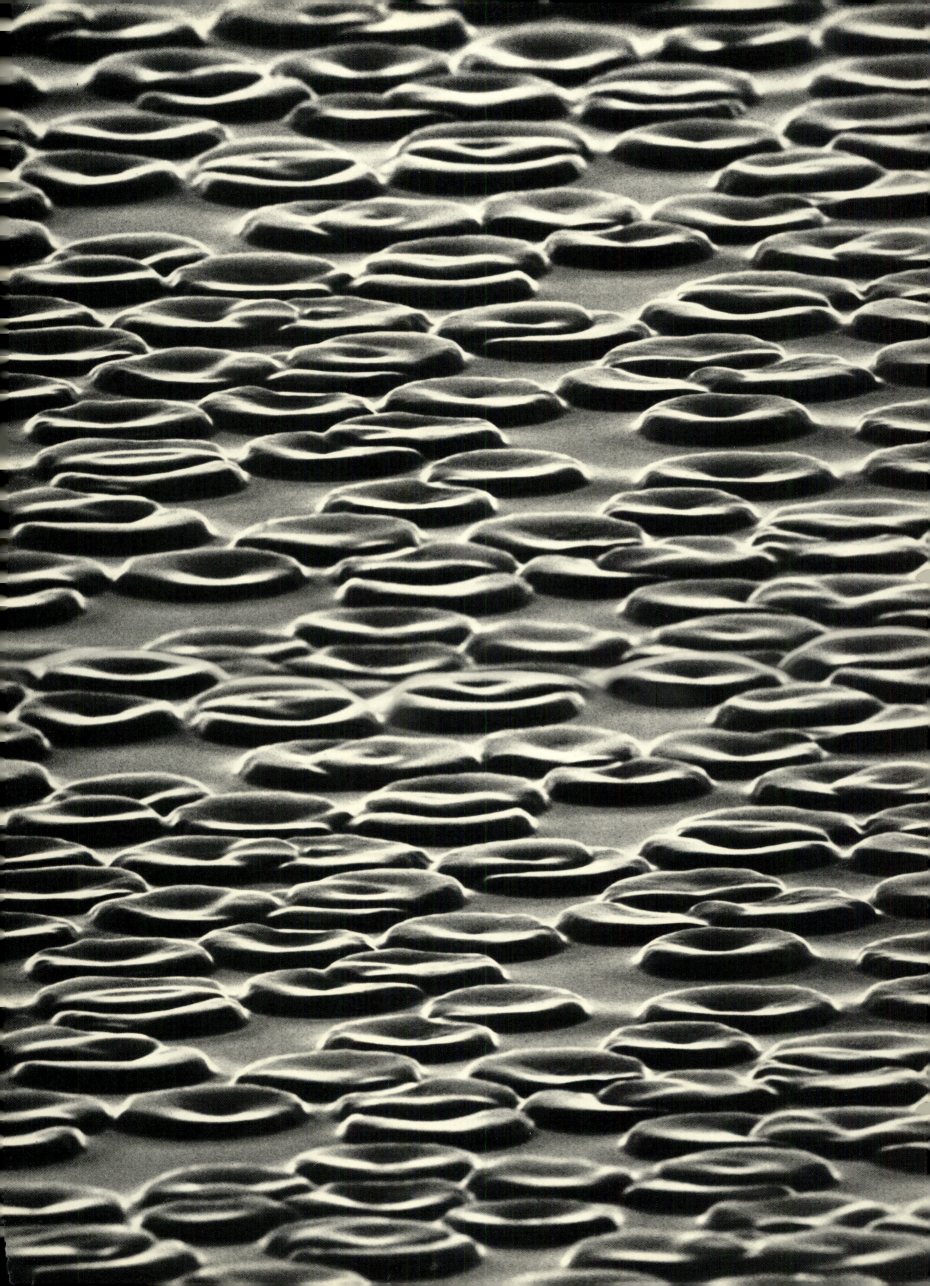

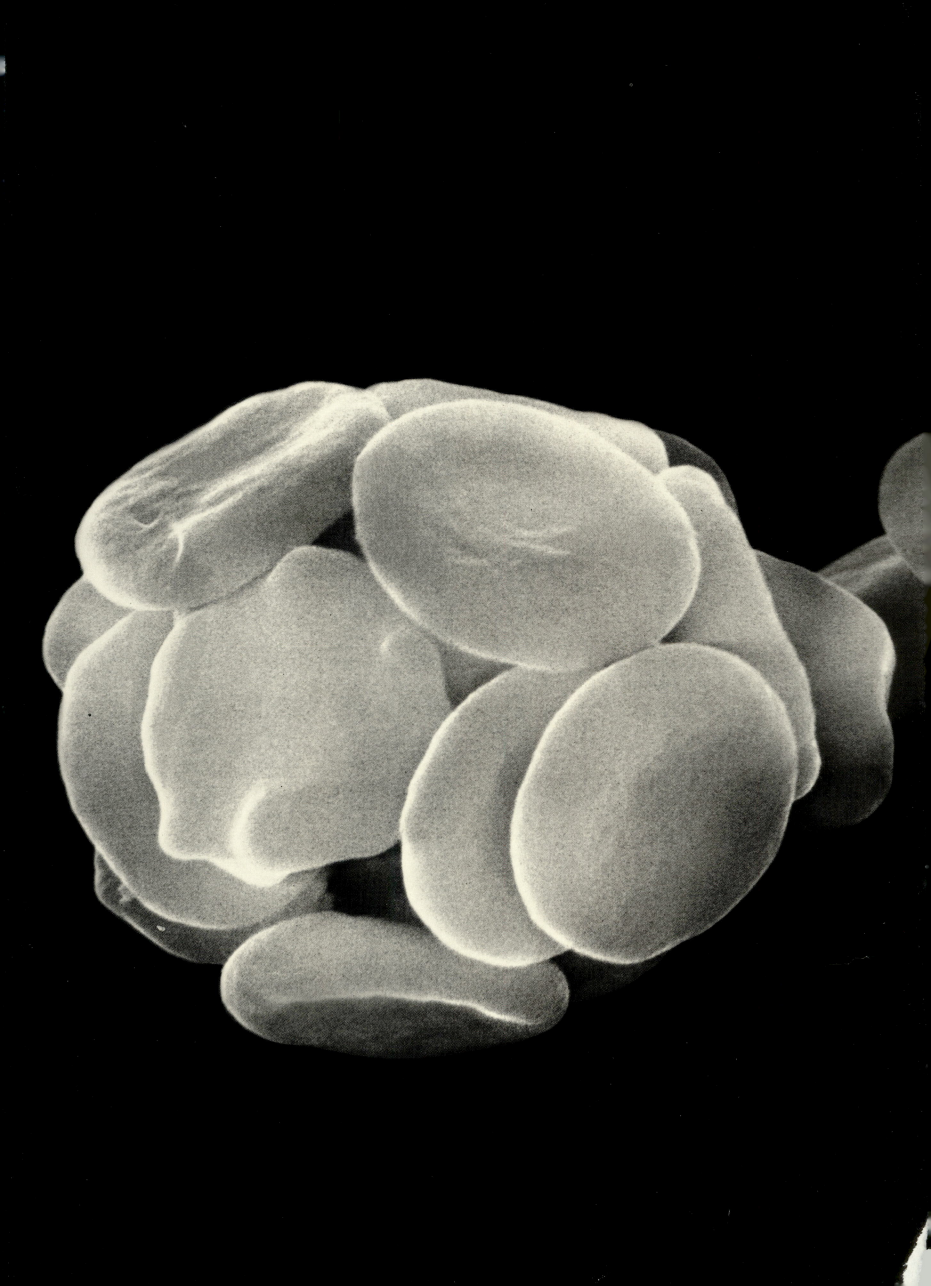

Chapter III

Echinocytes

Echinocytes

When red cells are washed in isotonic saline and observed between glass slide and coverslip, a transformation in their shape takes place. They change from a biconcave disc into a sphere covered with "spicules." This form is called a crenated cell or an Echinocyte. The phenomenon is due to the high pH induced by the glass. The transformation is reversible: when the same cells are washed with normal fresh plasma they resume their former discoid shape.

The echinocyte transformation can also be brought about by other extrinsic factors (such as lysolecithin or fatty acids) or by intrinsic factors (such as ATP depletion). Echinocytes appear after a few days when blood is preserved for transfusion. They return to their original disc form in the recipient's body.

It has been observed that the spicules always appear (or reappear) in the same place on the surface of the cell. No explanation has as yet been given for this phenomenon: the red cell membrane does not feature any special structures at these precise points (at least as far as we can now determine).

When red cells are exposed to high concentrations of echinocytic agents, they become more spherical, and the spicules become very fine needle-like projections. These forms are called sphero-echinocytes.

Fig. 1. Two discocytes and an echinocyte.

Figs. 2 to 7. Progressive transformation of discocyte into echinocyte. An echinocyte I is an irregularly contoured discocyte. An echinocyte II is a flat red cell with spicules. An echinocyte III is an ovoid or spherical cell with 30 to 40 spicules evenly distributed over its surface.

Figs. 8 and 9. Comparison between a normal and an inverted echinocyte.

Fig. 10. Mixture of discocytes and sphero-echinocytes. Blood from a normal individual was separated into two parts; one immediately fixed, the other exposed for 10 minutes to sodium oleate, in order to obtain sphero-echinocytes, then the two parts were mixed. The cell volumes remained unchanged.

Fig. 11. Echinocyte II. A single spicule has formed in the center.

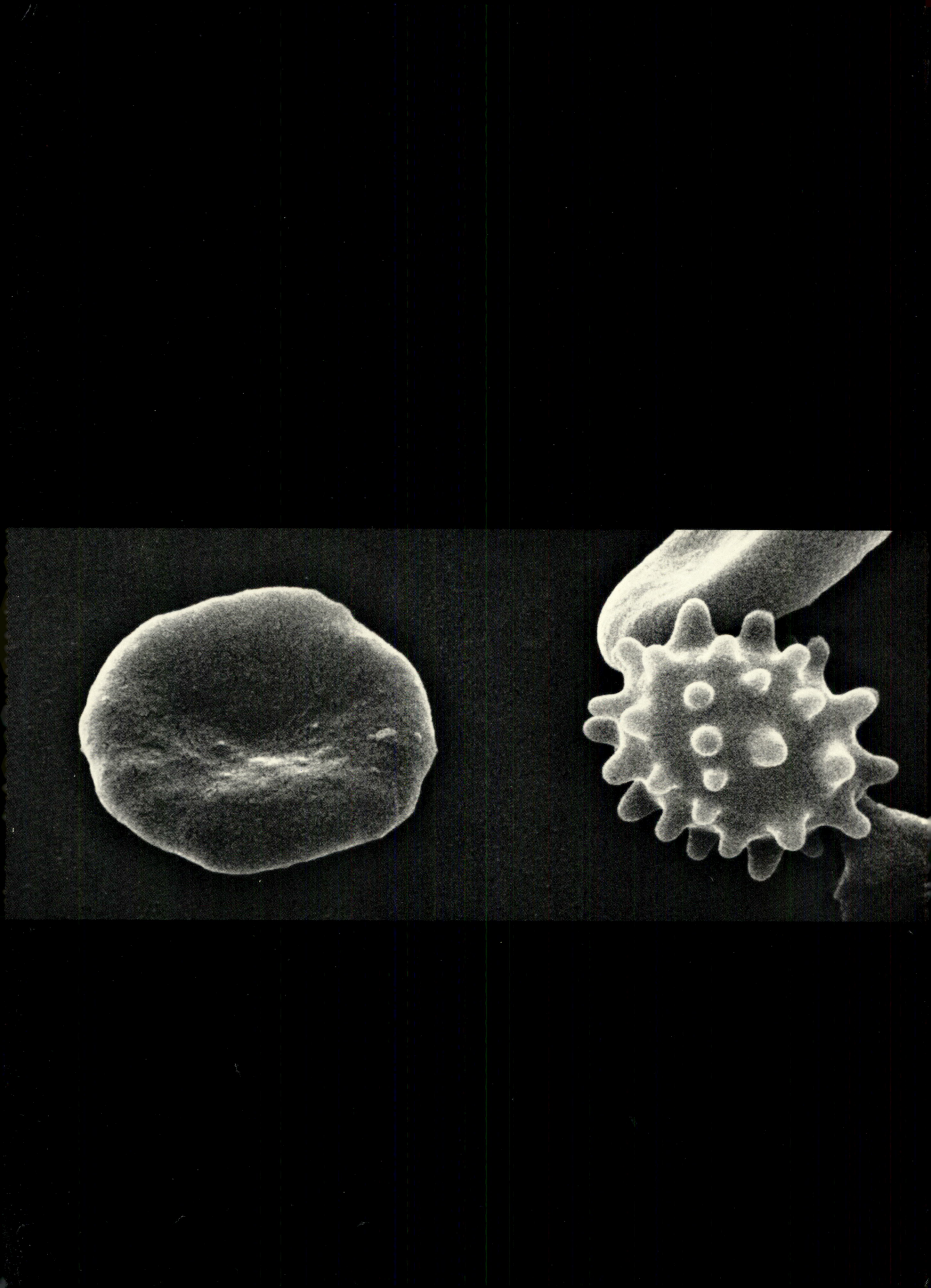

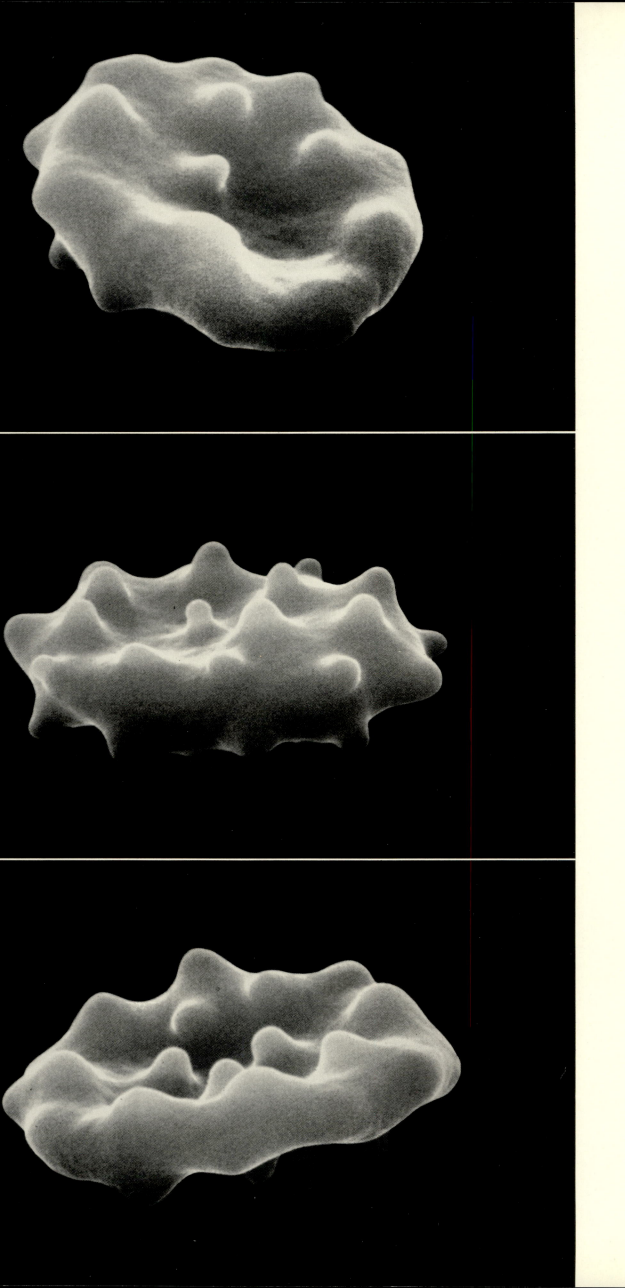

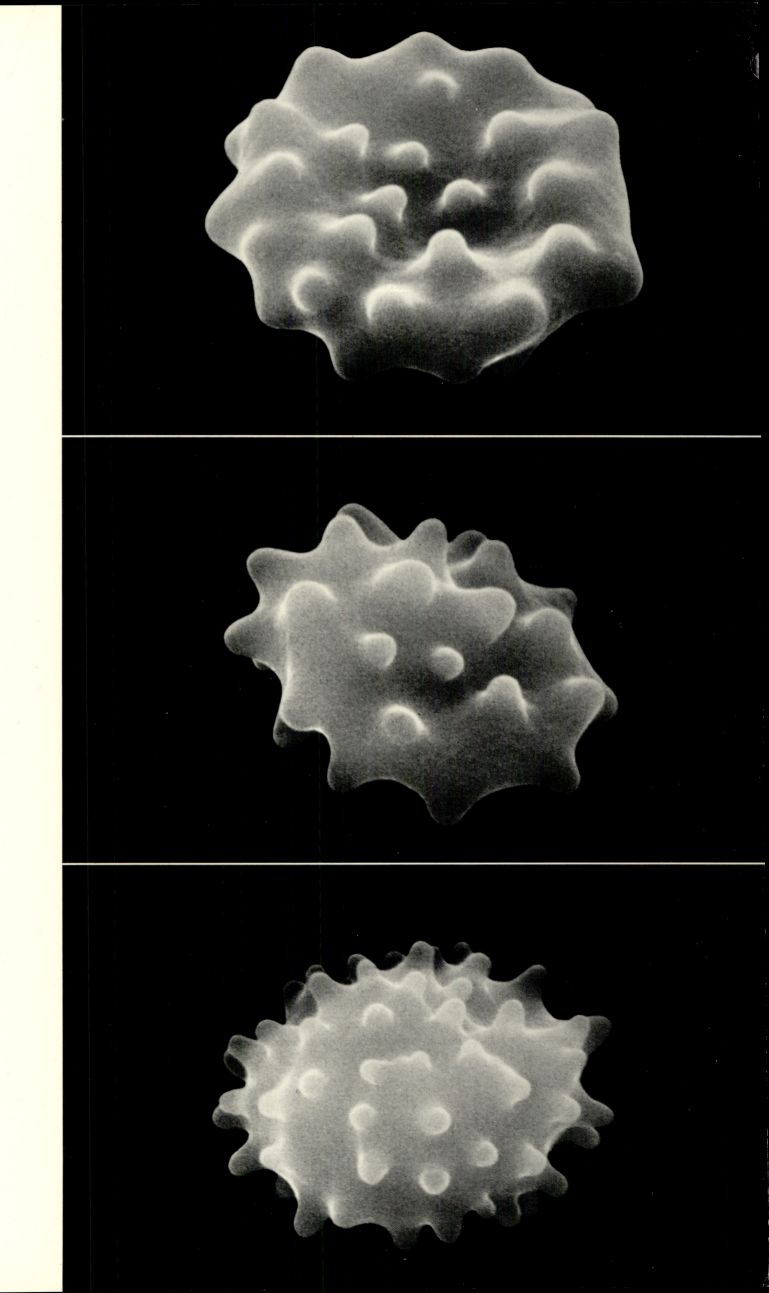

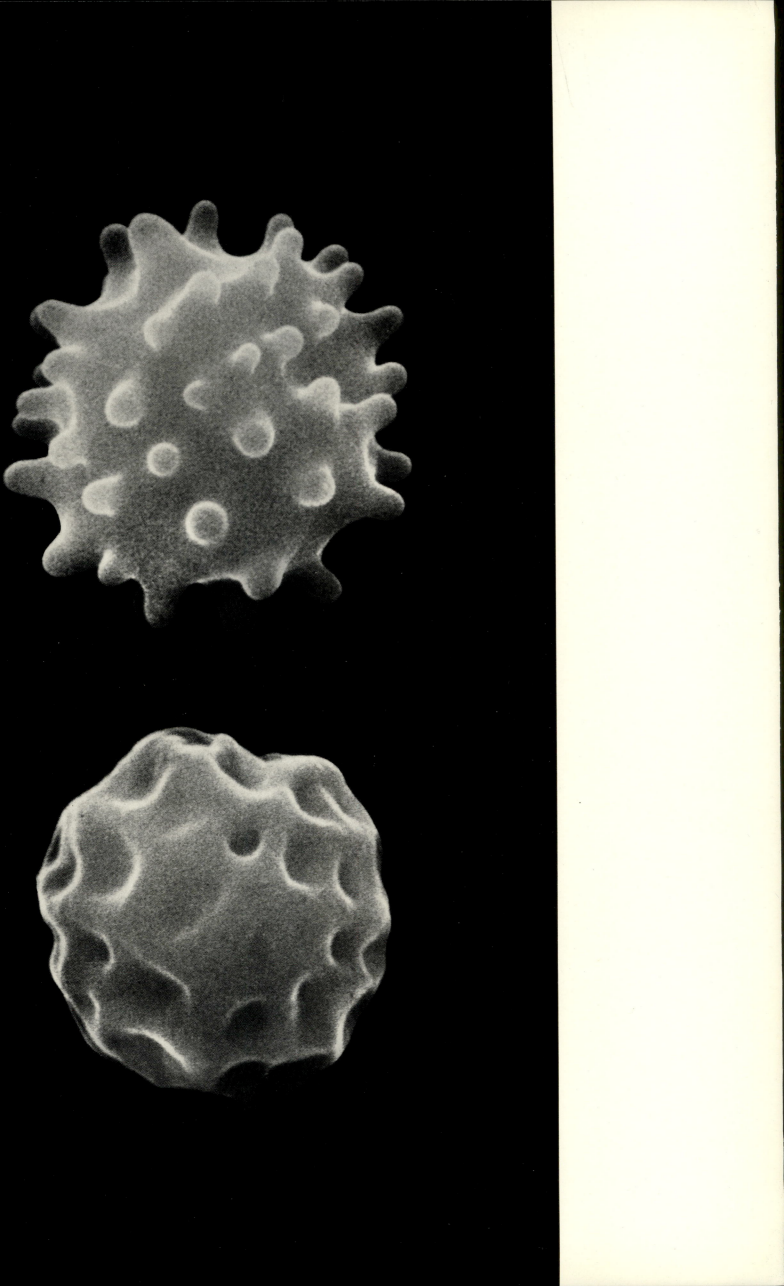

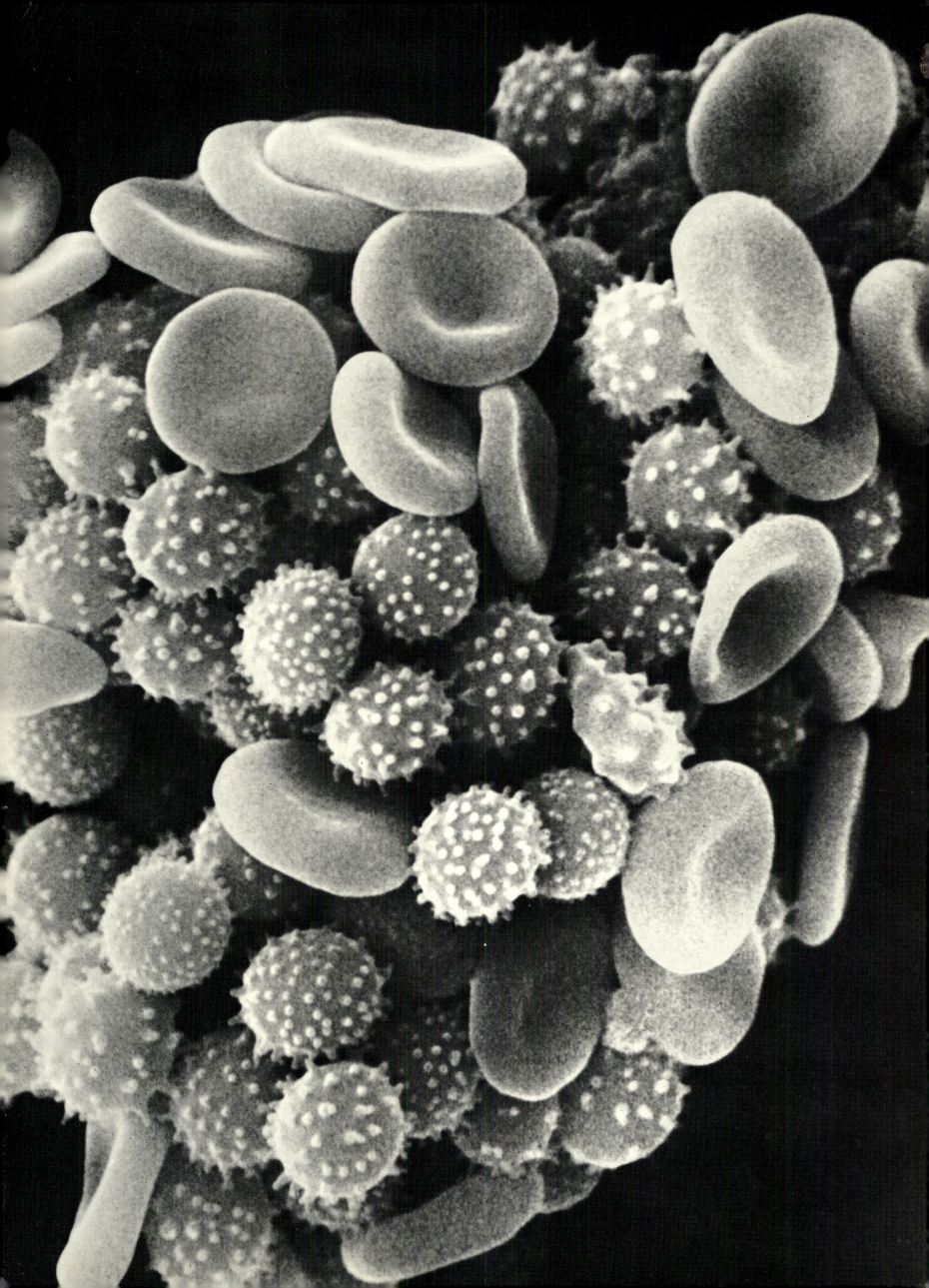

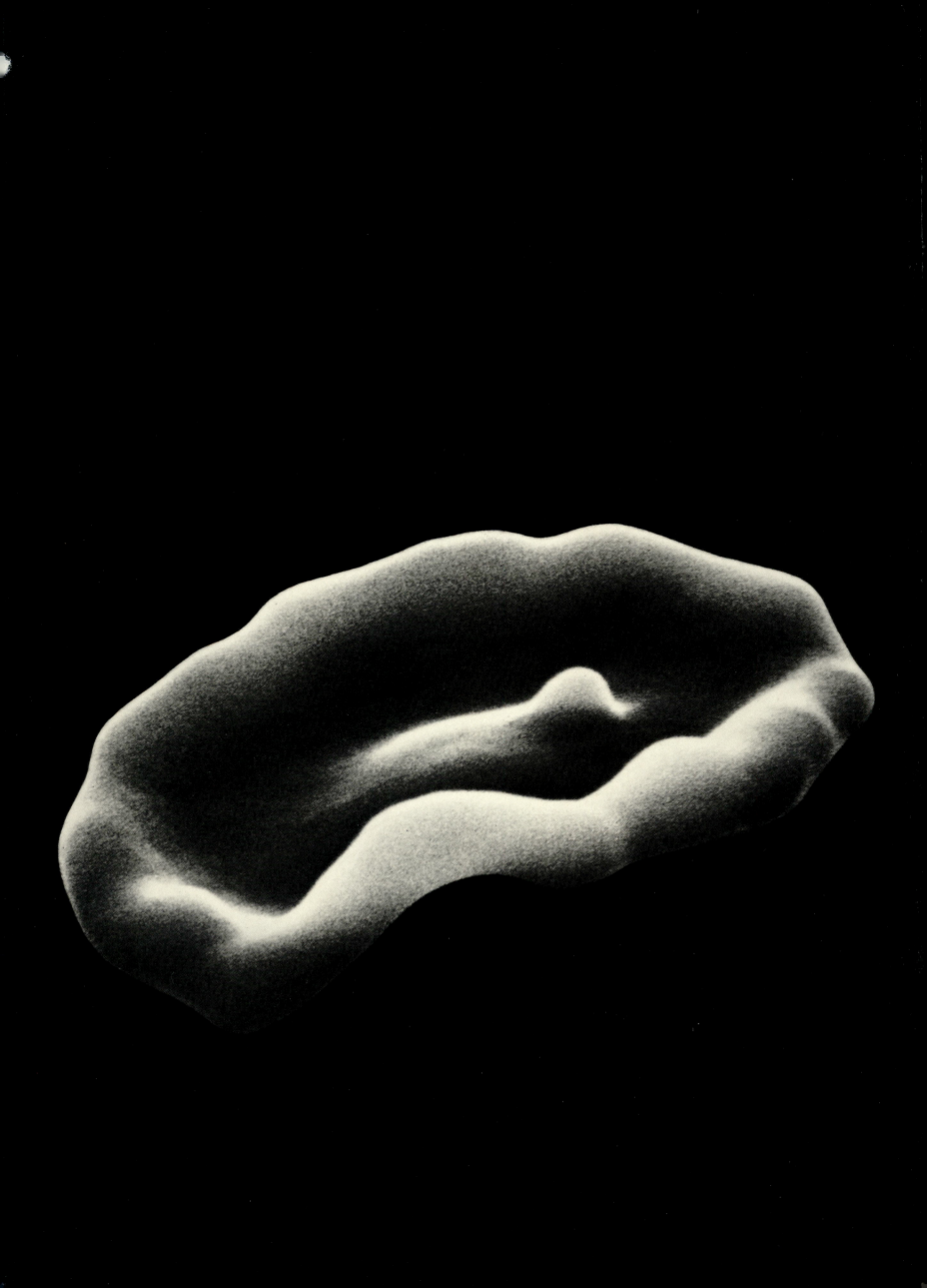

Chapter IV

Stomatocytes

Stomatocytes

The stomatocytic transformation is the converse of the echinocytic transformation. Rather than everted spicules, there is an inverted mouth. Low pH and chemical agents (e.g. phenothiazines) produce cup-like cells. These are called "stomatocytes" (from the Greek word meaning mouth), since the inversion frequently appears (particularly when flattened on a smear) as an elongated depression edged by two lips.

When red cells are exposed to high concentrations of stomatocytic agents, they become more spherical, and the mouth shrinks to a dimple. These forms are called "stomato-spherocytes."

Although there is a resemblance between echino-spheres and stomato-spheres in their final spherical stages, the scanning electron microscope easily detects the remnants of spicules or of a dimple.

Like the discocyte-echinocyte transformation, the disco-stomatocyte transformation may occur in pathological erythrocytes. This transformation is superimposed upon the underlying structural pathology of the cell. We will return to this phenomenon in later chapters.

Fig. 1. Stomatocyte. This name comes from the Greek word for mouth.

Figs. 2, 3 and 4. Progressive transformation of a stomatocyte into a spherostomatocyte. Note the irregular area on the left side of the cell (Fig. 4).

Fig. 5. Stomatocytes I and II.

Fig. 6. Sphero-stomatocyte II. This cell was obtained by the action of phenothiazine.

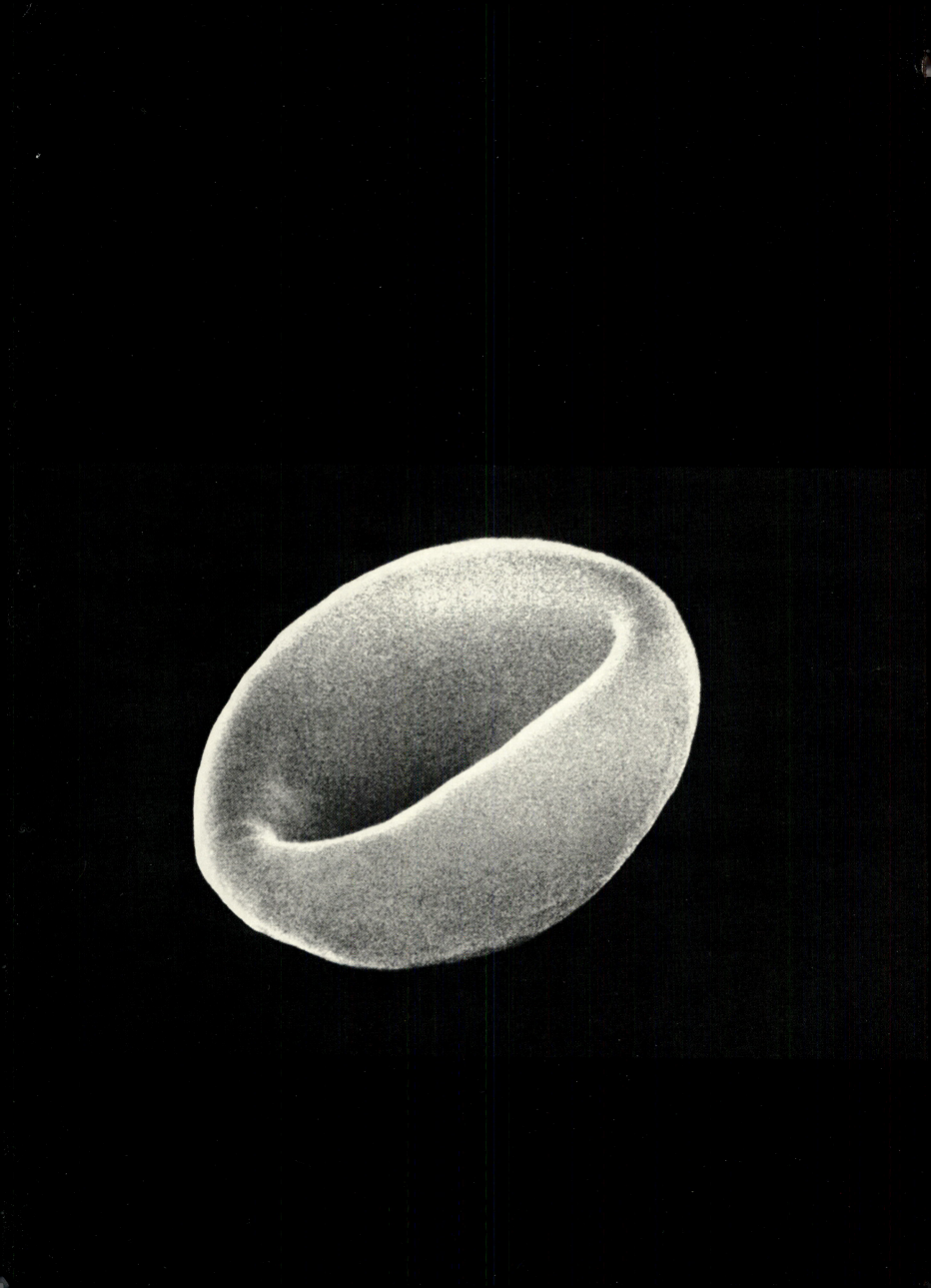

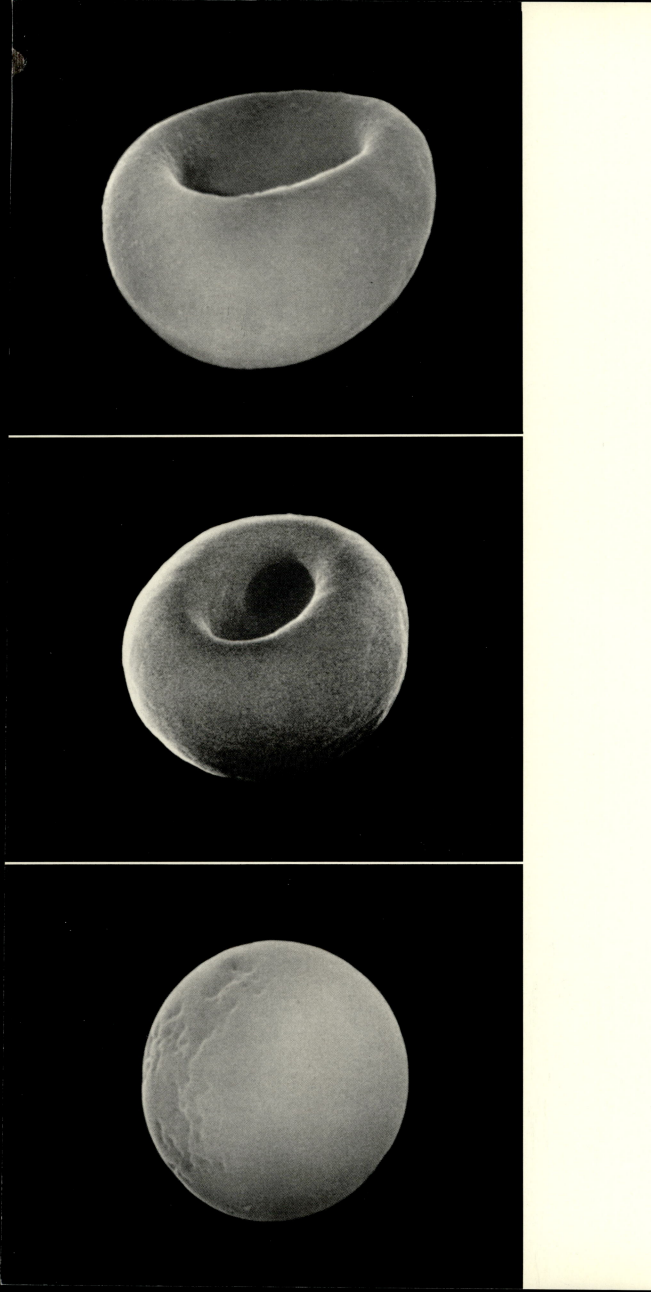

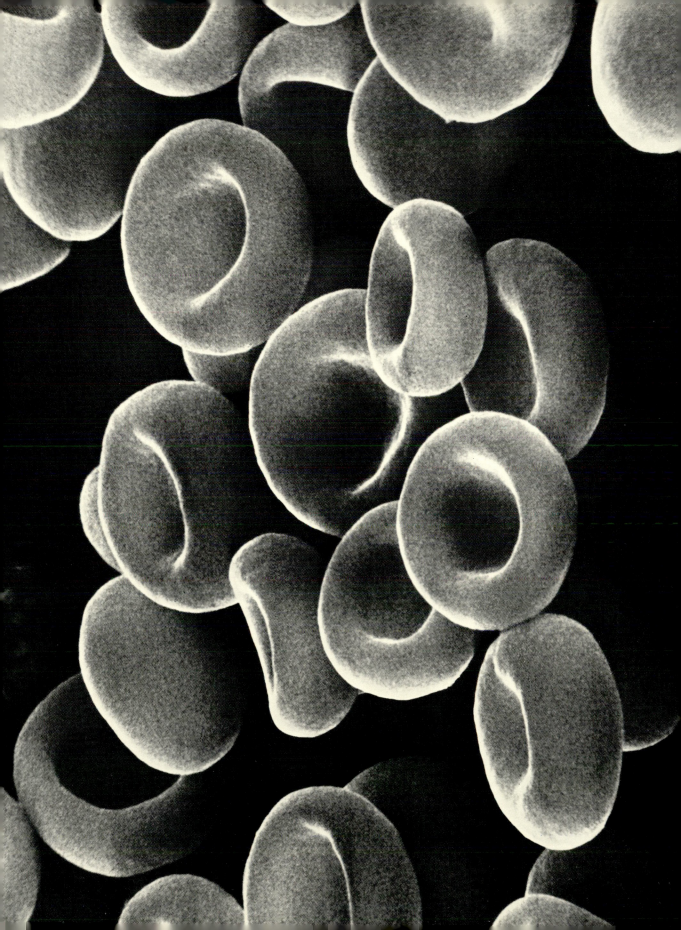

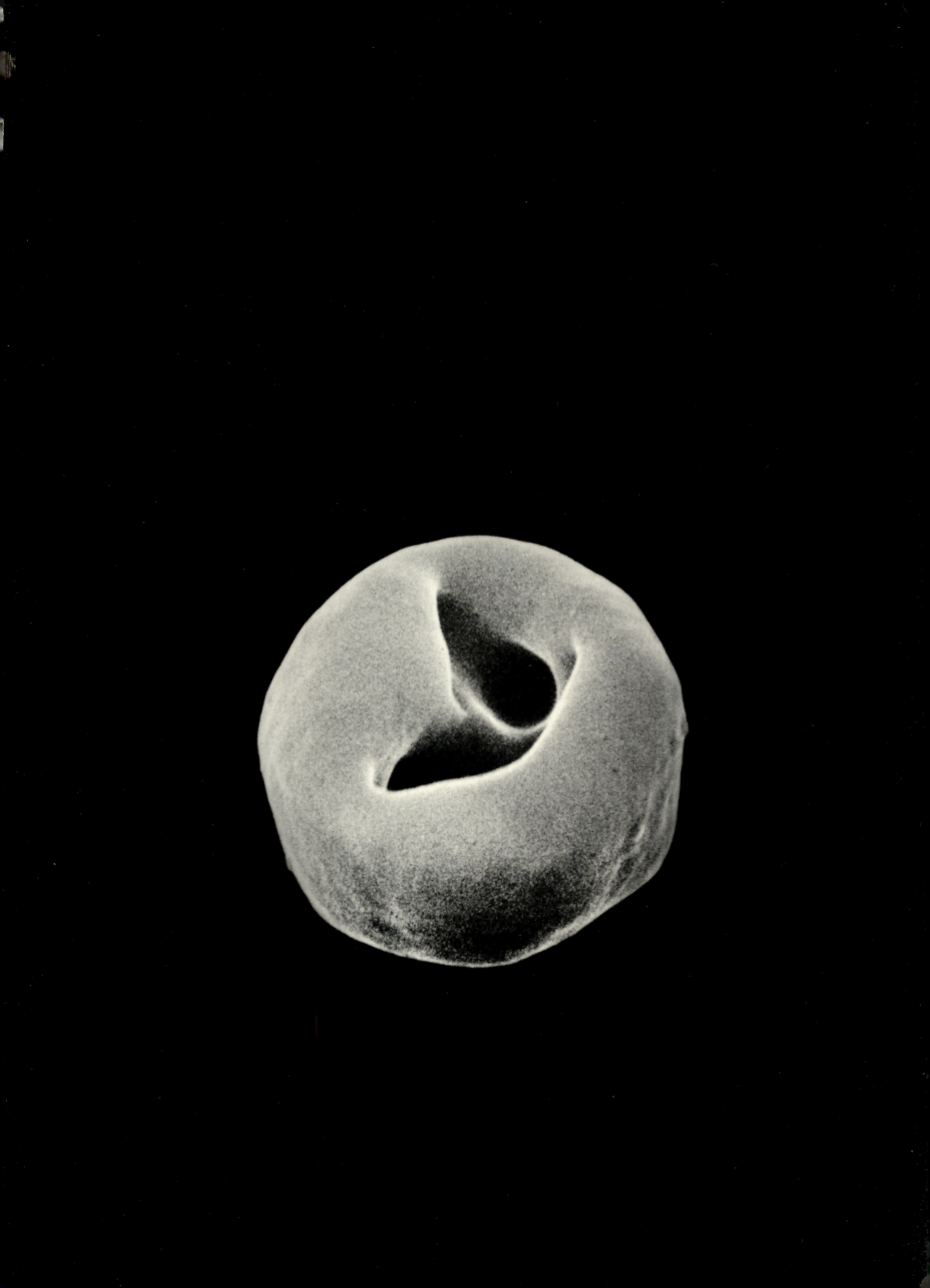

Chapter V

Drepanocytes

Drepanocytes

Drepanocytosis (or sickle cell anemia) is a hereditary disease which is largely confined to black people. In the red cells of patients who suffer from this condition, normal hemoglobin (A) is replaced by an abnormal hemoglobin (S). When the oxygen tension decreases (for instance at high altitude), the hemoglobin molecules polymerize and form tiny, long rods inside the cell. These small rods of hemoglobin cluster into sheaf-like bundles which stretch the membrane and deform the discocyte. Such cells appear sickle-shaped.

Sickle cells are rigid and cause dramatic alterations in the viscosity and flow properties of blood. In the circulation, they block blood flow in narrow capillaries, causing stasis and poor oxygen supply to the tissues, and finally painful abdominal crises, splenic infarcts or cerebral and renal damage. Sickle cells are mechanically fragile: their long spicules can break, leading to hemolysis of the cell.

Fig. 1. Drepanocyte, or sickle cell, developed from an SS discocyte.

Figs. 2, 3, and 4. Different aspects of drepanocytes.

Fig. 5. Drepanocyte with many spikes. Note how they all develop in a single plane (compare with the drepano-echinocyte in the next chapter).

Figs. 6 and 7. Drepanocytes with spikes covering the entire circumference of the cell ("holly-leaf" cell: such forms can also occur when S hemoglobin polymerizes in an echinocyte I.)

Figs. 8 and 9. Two long-armed drepanocytes.

Fig. 10. Drepanocyte and drepano-echinocyte I.

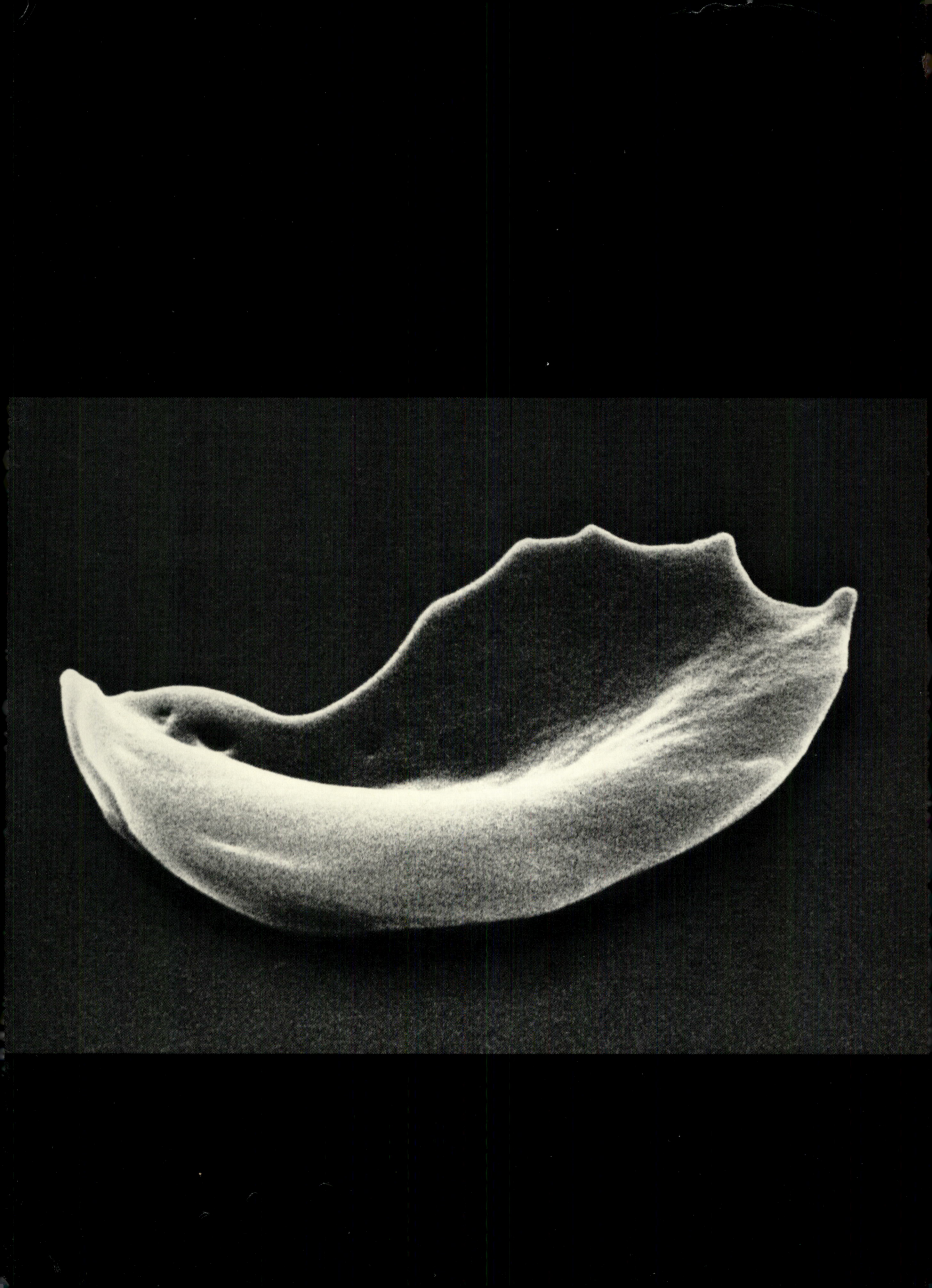

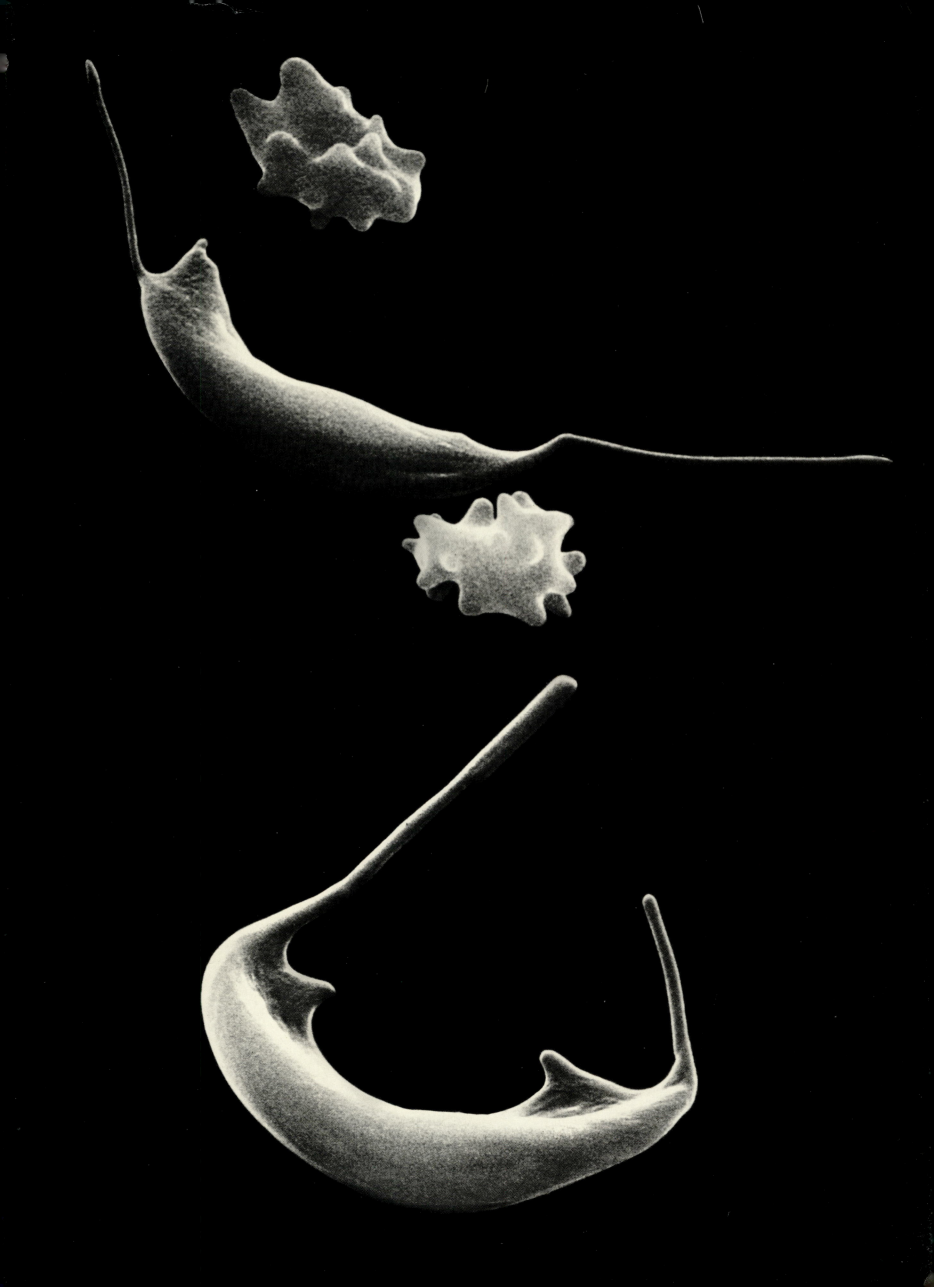

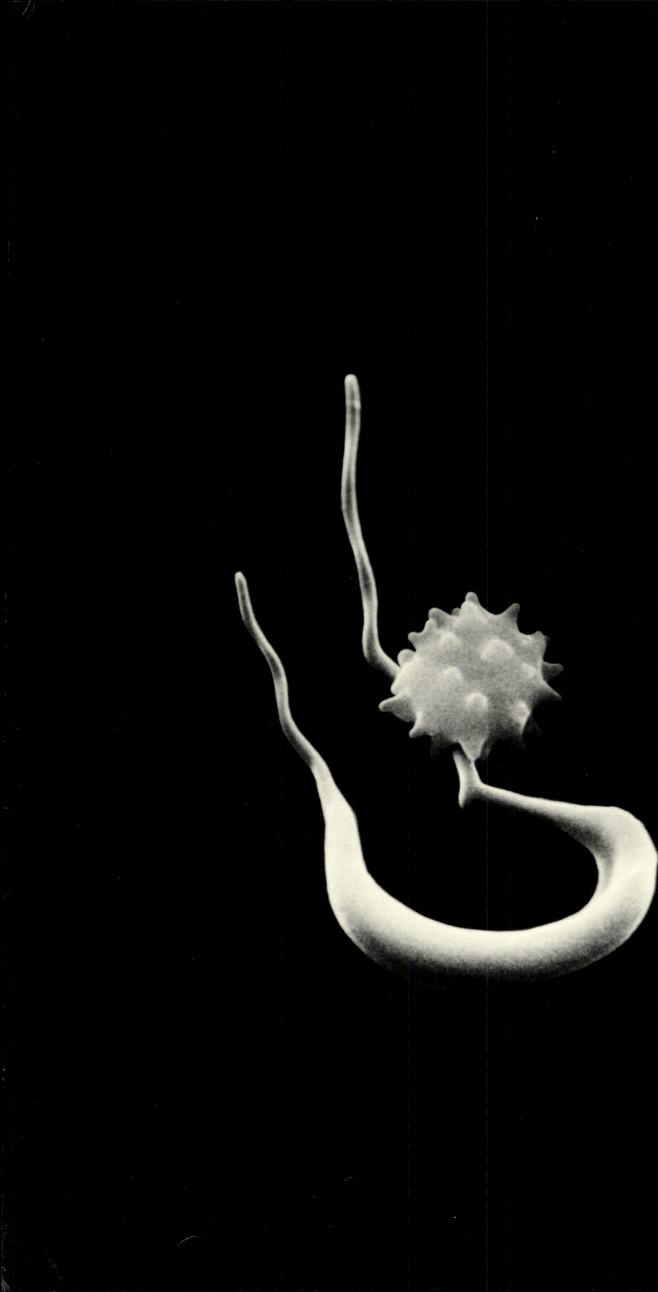

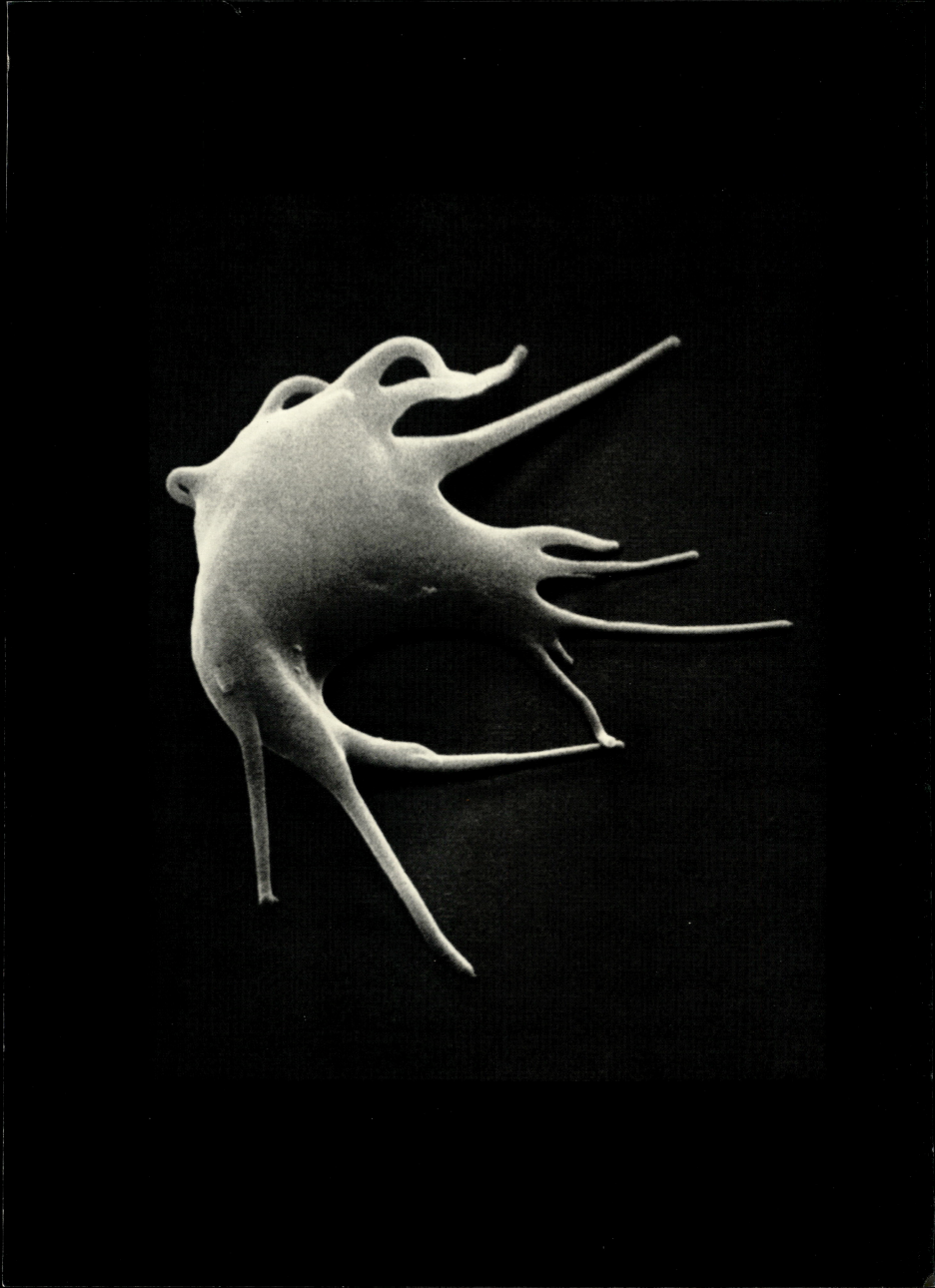

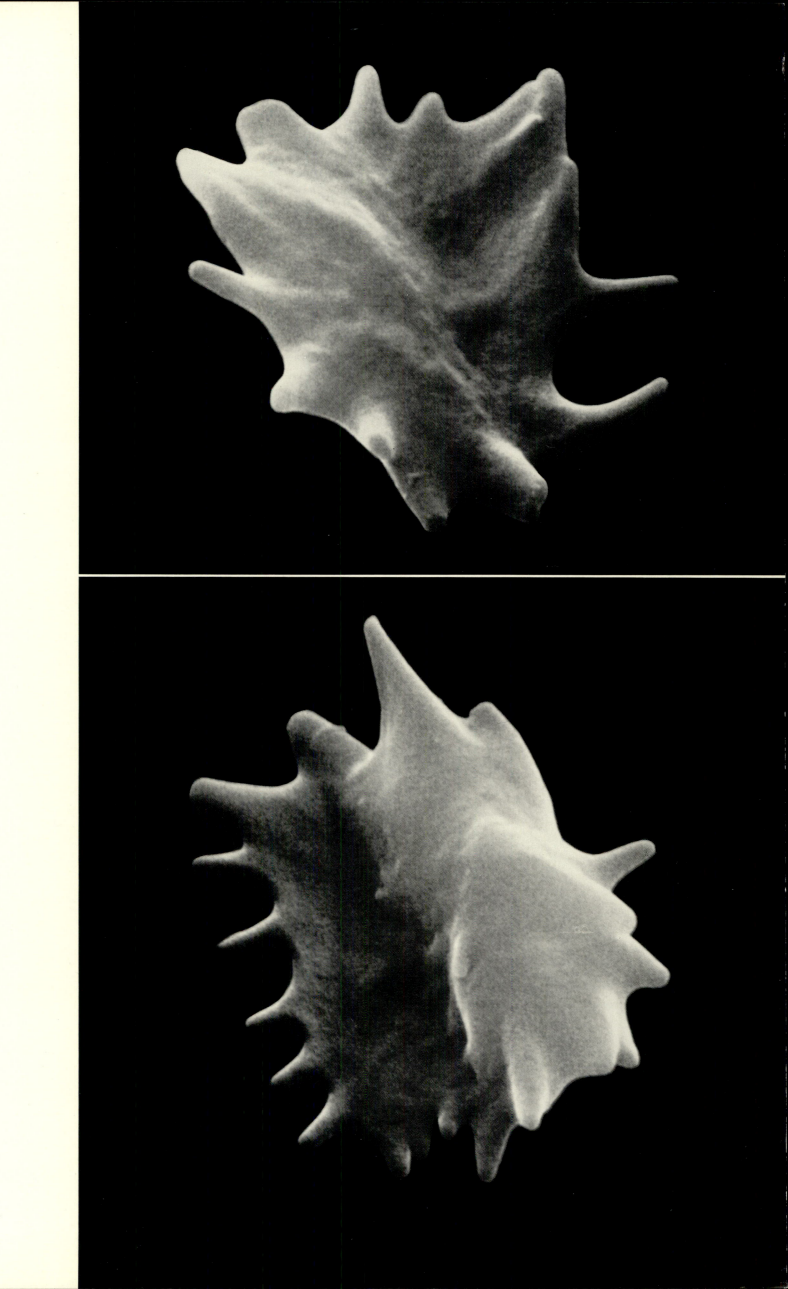

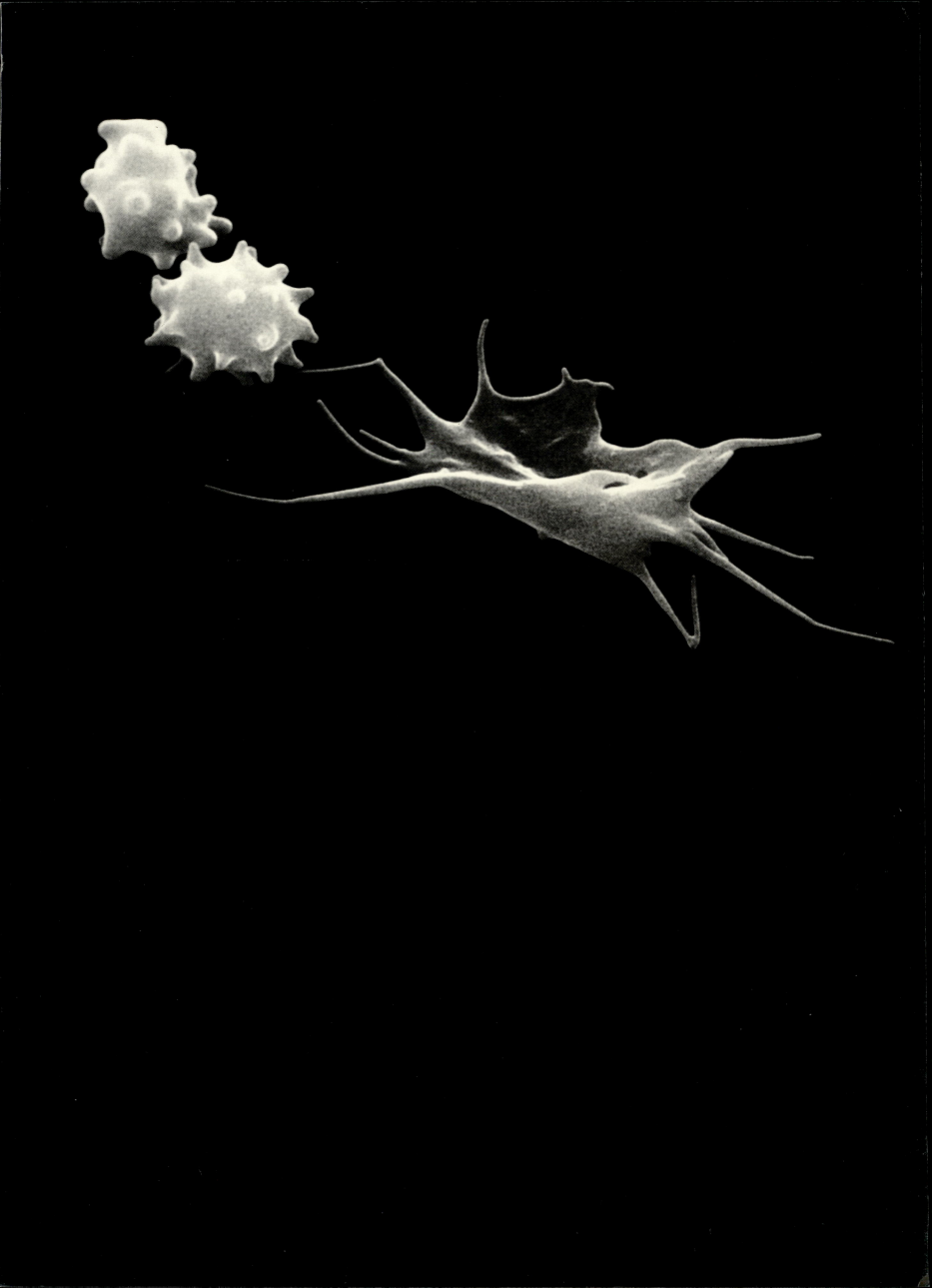

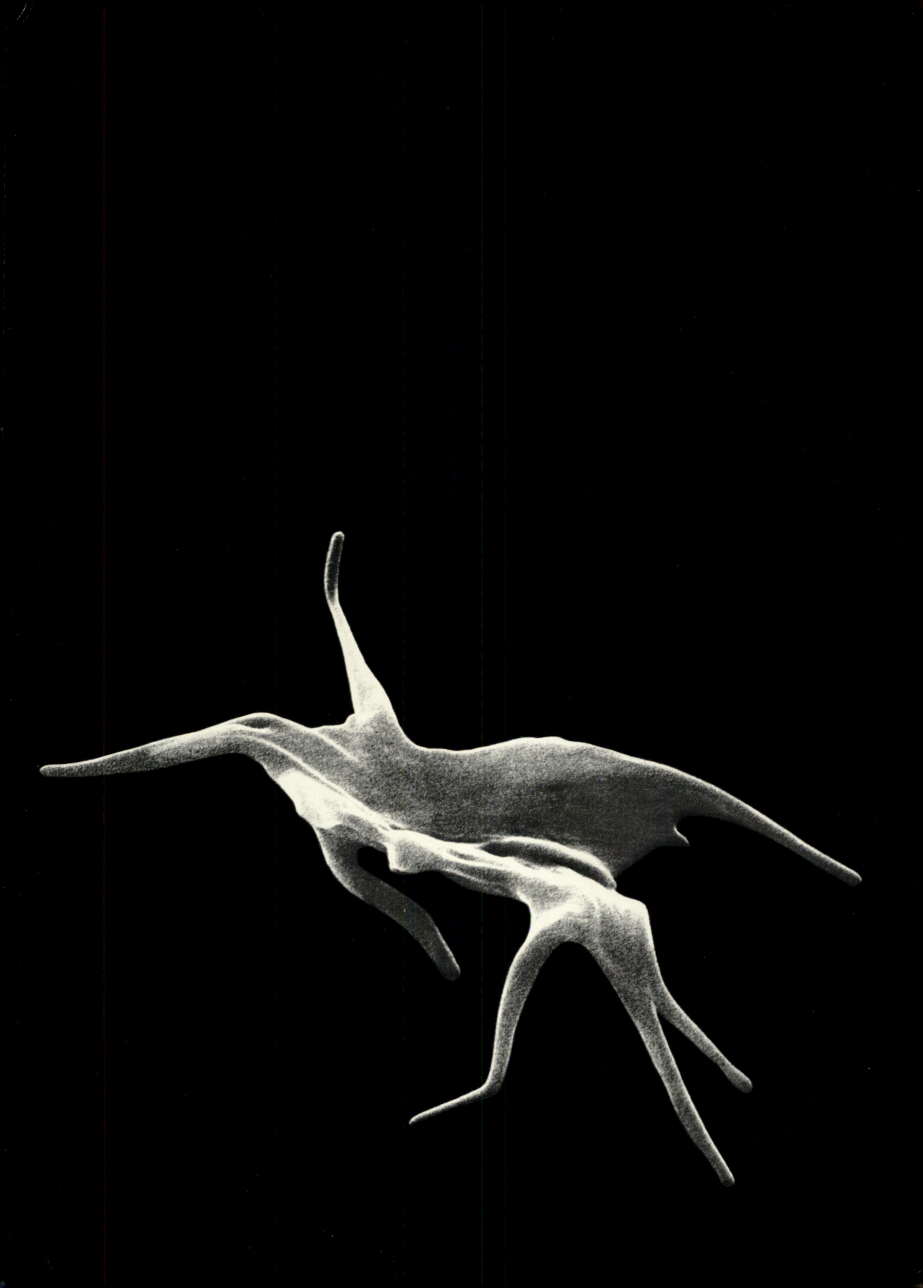

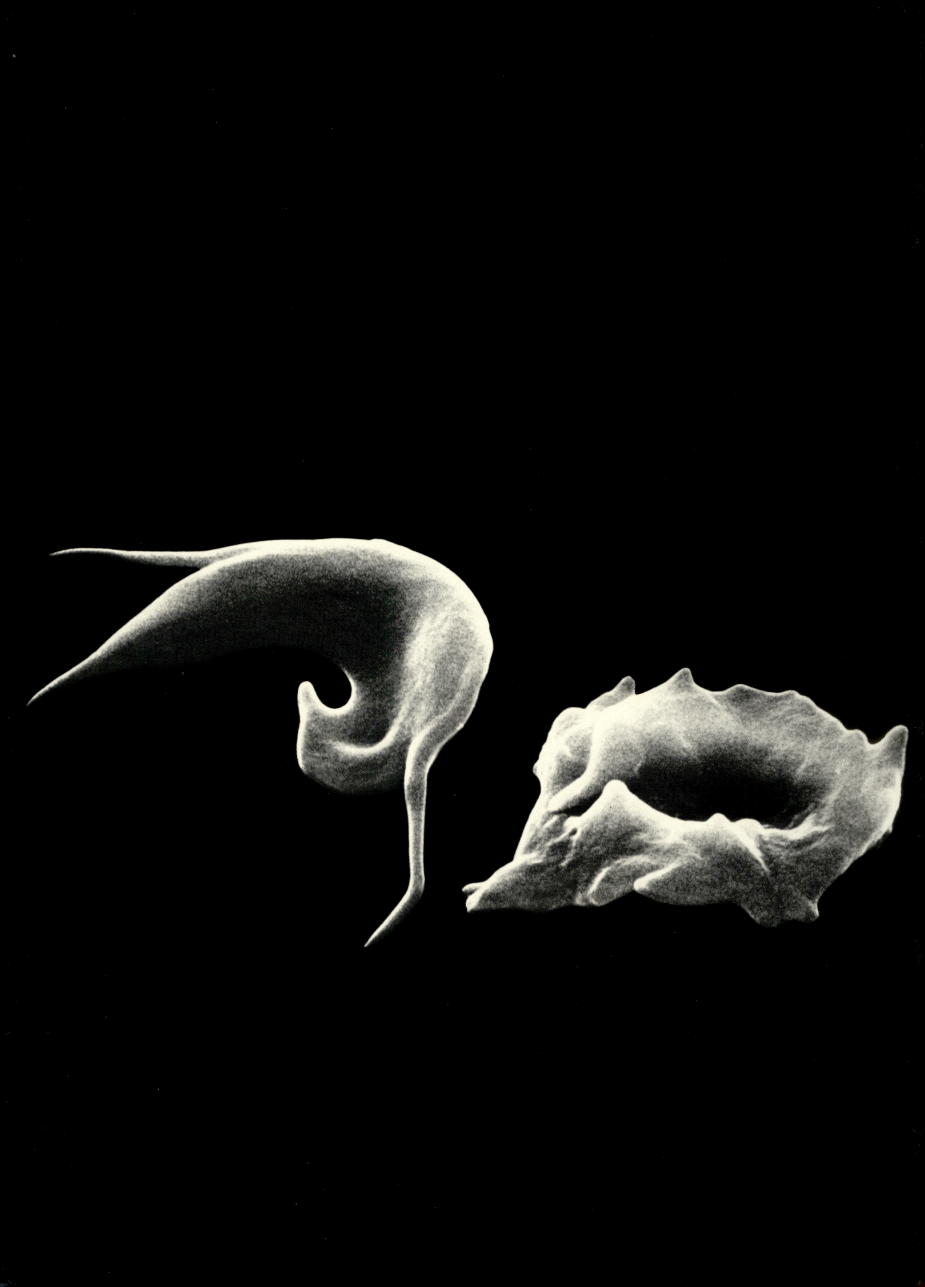

Chapter VI

Echino-Drepanocytes and Stomato-Drepanocytes

Echino-Drepanocytes
and Stomato-Drepanocytes

Discocytes containing S hemoglobin can, like normal erythrocytes, undergo the echinocytic, or stomatocytic, transformation.

In S-echinocytes, reduced oxygen tension leads to polymerization of the S hemoglobin. In an echinocyte I, which is still disc-shaped, the stiff hemoglobin rods stretch out at the rim of the disc and a holly-leaf appearance results. In echinocytes II and III, the hemoglobin rods develop in all three dimensions and a rigid echinocyte results in which the individual spicules, unchanged in number and location, have become remarkably elongated and are of uneven length. The initially round or pointed tips of the individual spicules assume the appearance of truncated cones.

If the oxygen tension is reduced in an S-stomatocyte, the rods of polymerized hemoglobin spread along the inner surface of the membrane and follow its general contour. The cell becomes deformed and rigid, while retaining its overall cup-shaped appearance.

Fig. 1. Drepano-echinocyte. Initial treatment with sodium oleate (to make the cell echinocytic) followed by treatment with sodium metabisulfite (to remove the oxygen and let the hemoglobin polymerize).

Fig. 2. Drepano-stomatocyte. Initial treatment with chloropromazine (to make the cell stomatocytic) followed by treatment with sodium metabisulfite.

Figs. 3 and 4. Drepano-echinocytes.

Fig. 5. Drepano-echinocytes. The rods have developed within the echinocyte spicules.

Fig. 6. Drepano-stomatocyte. The spikes have developed at the edge of the cup.

Fig. 7. Drepano-echinocytes. A bizarre collection.

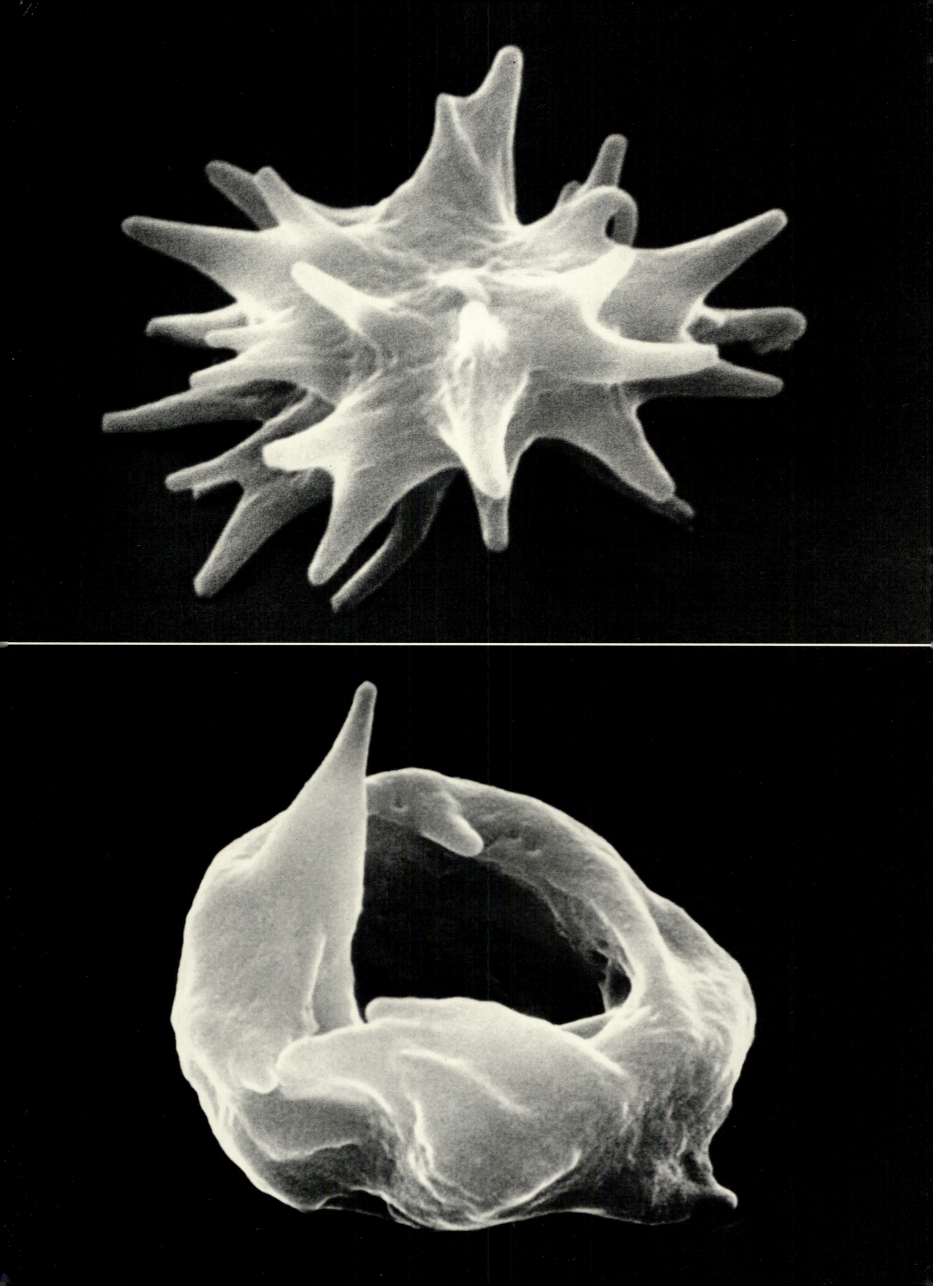

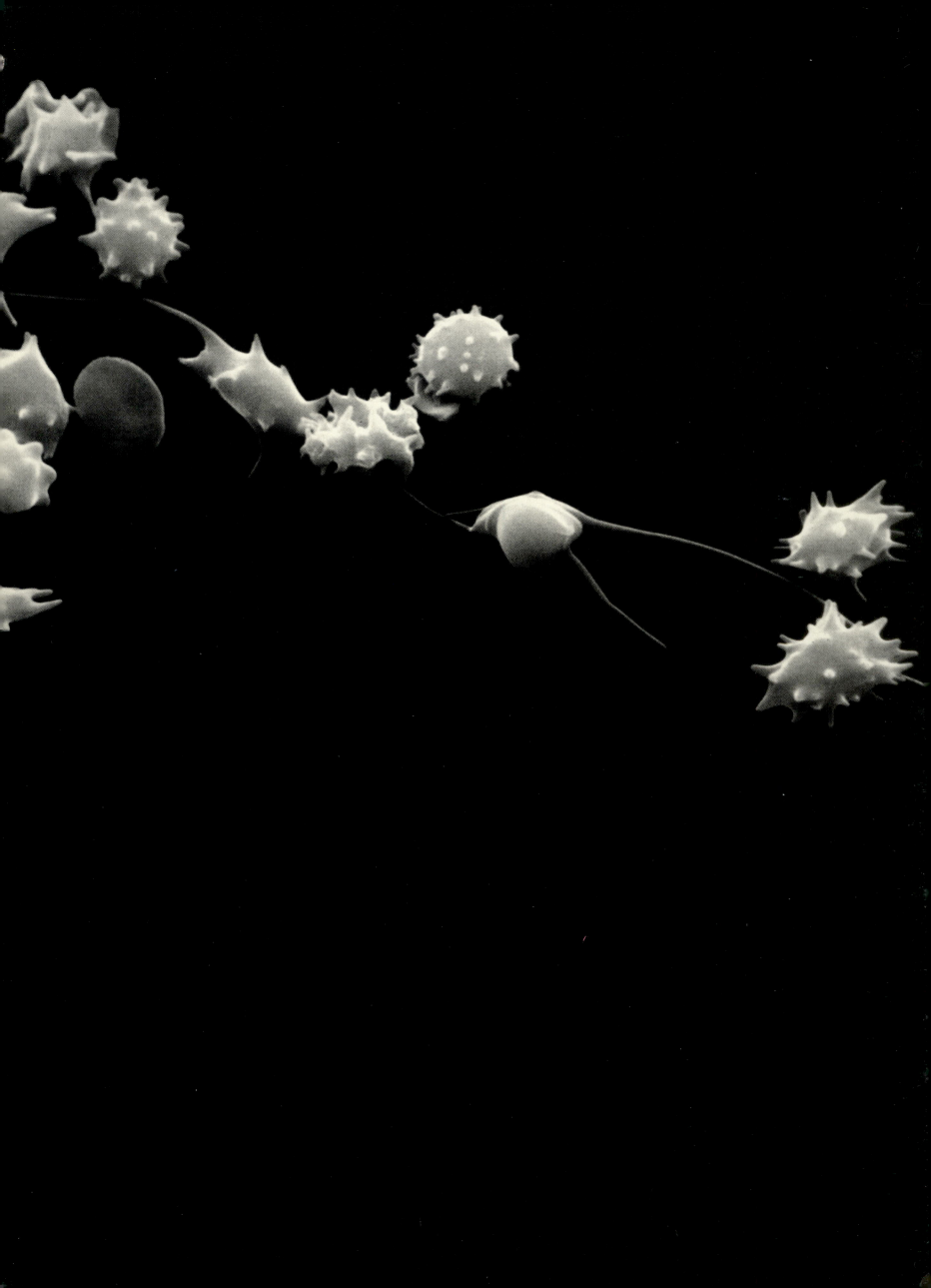

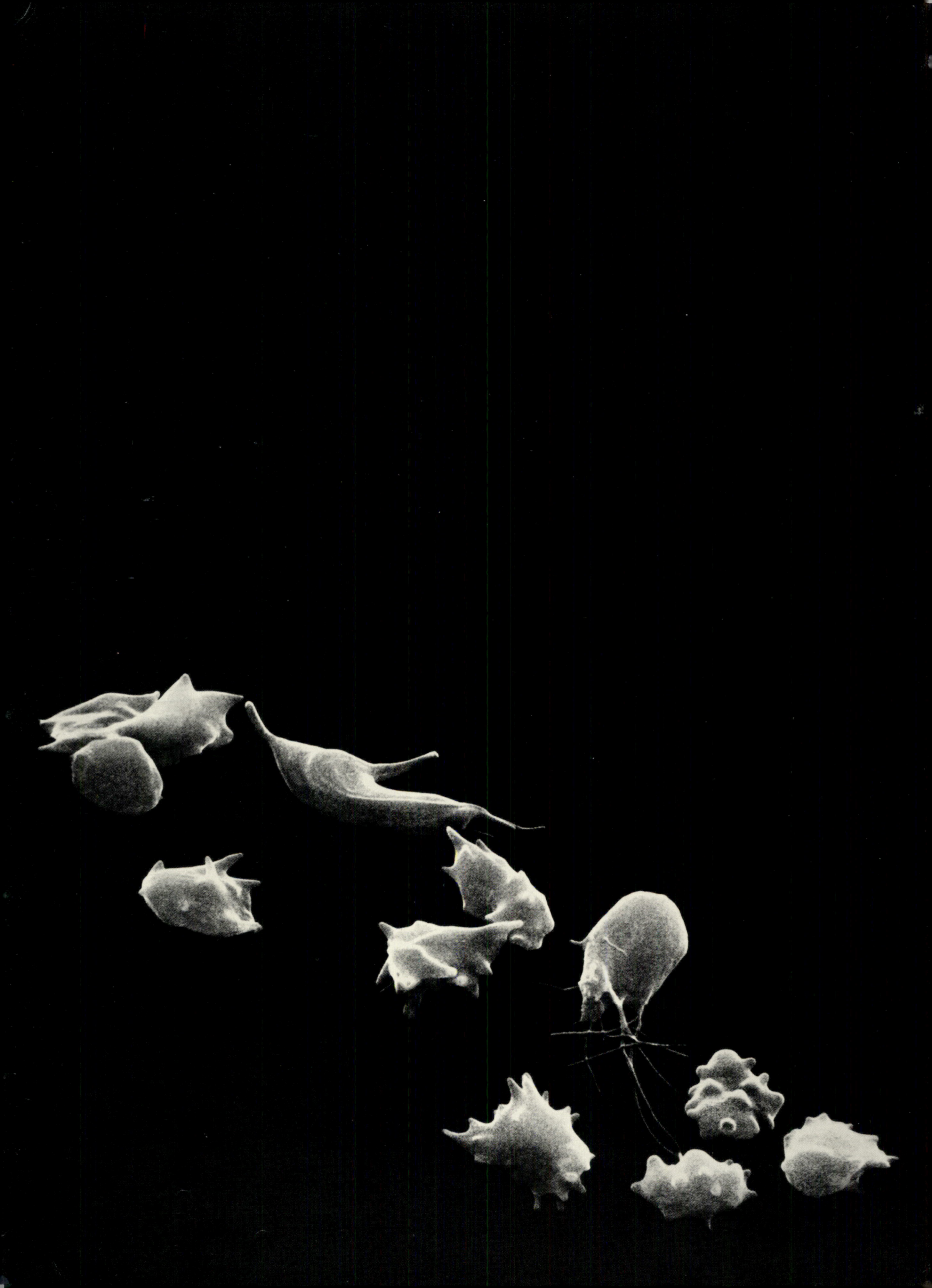

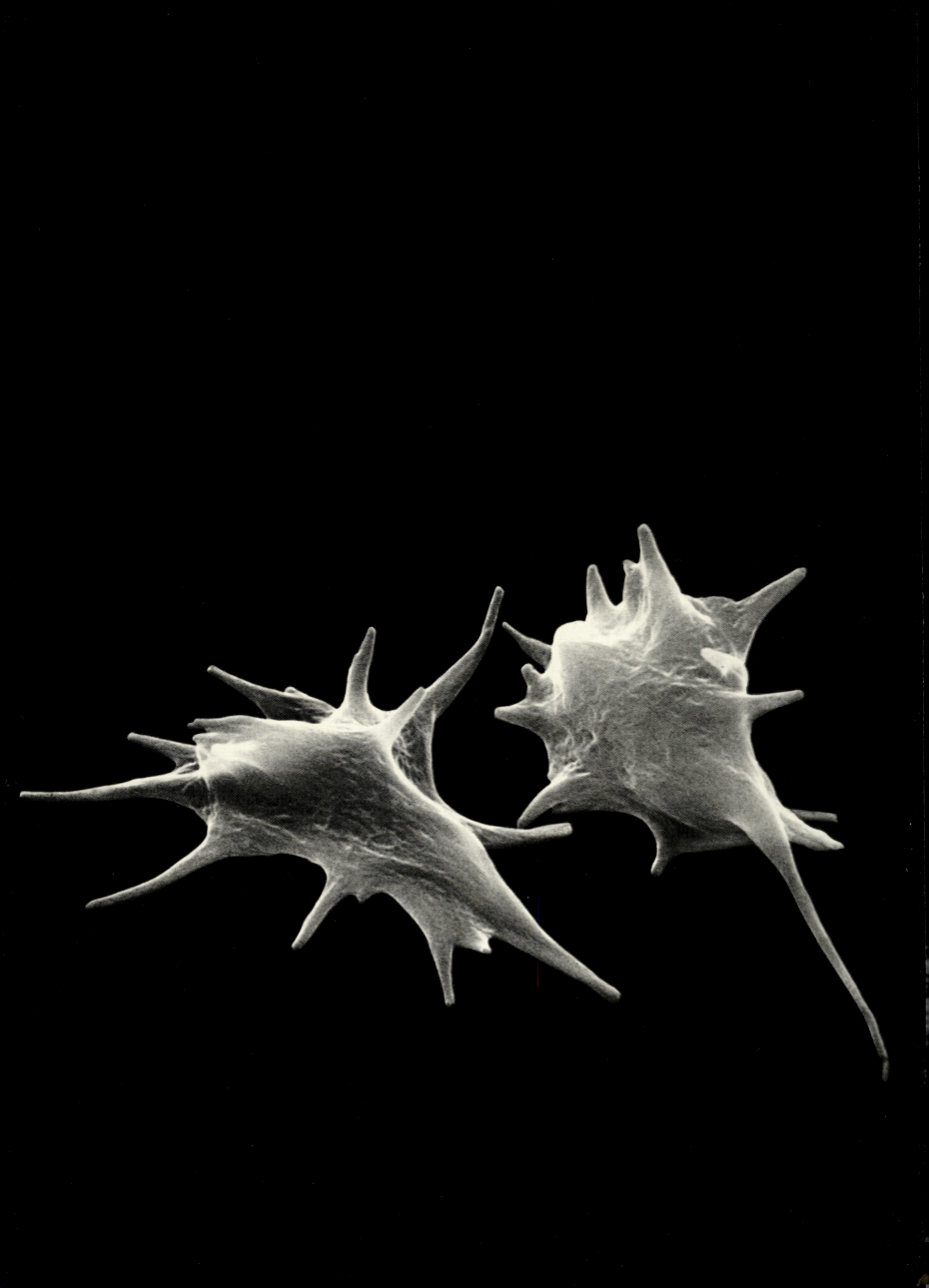

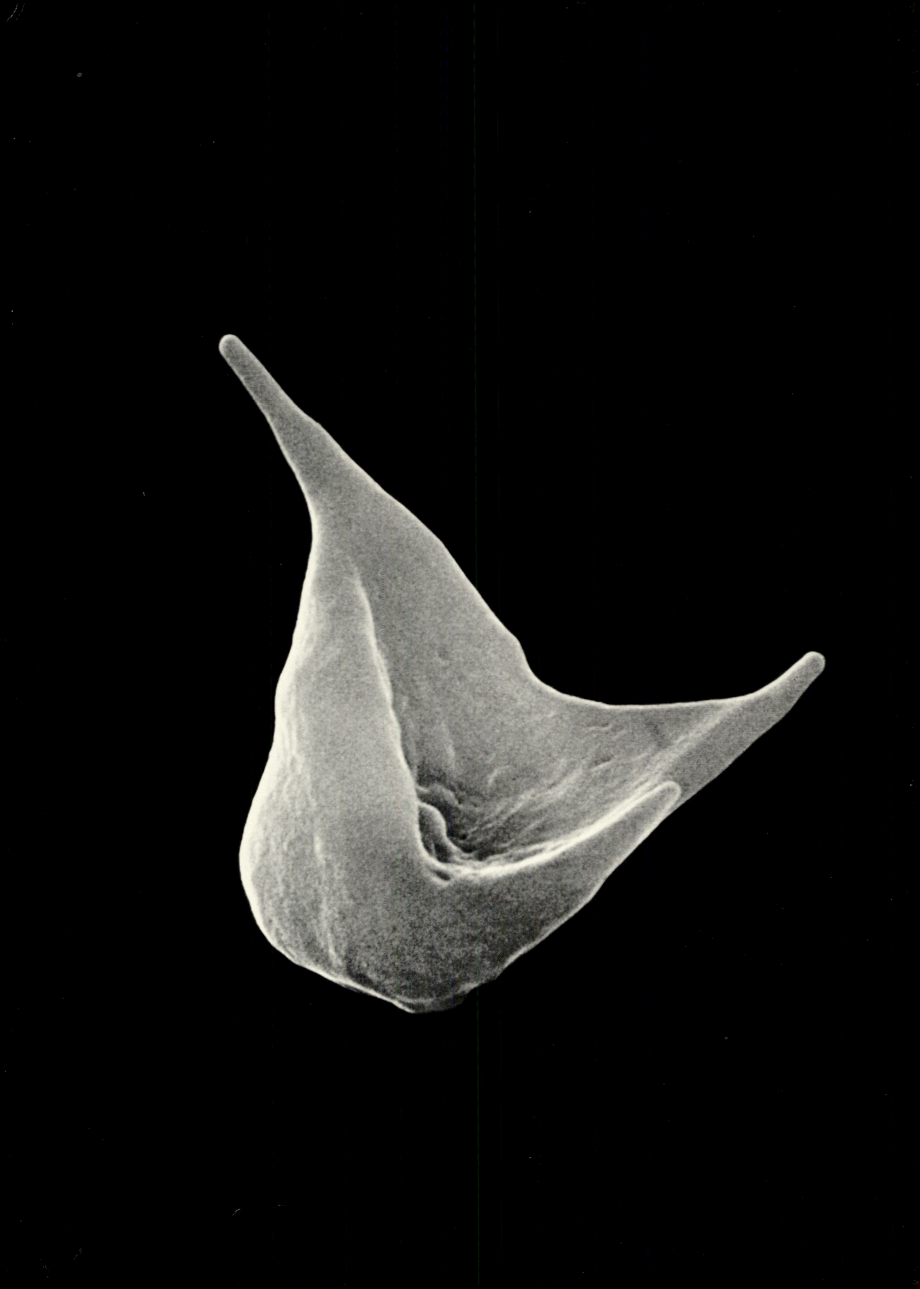

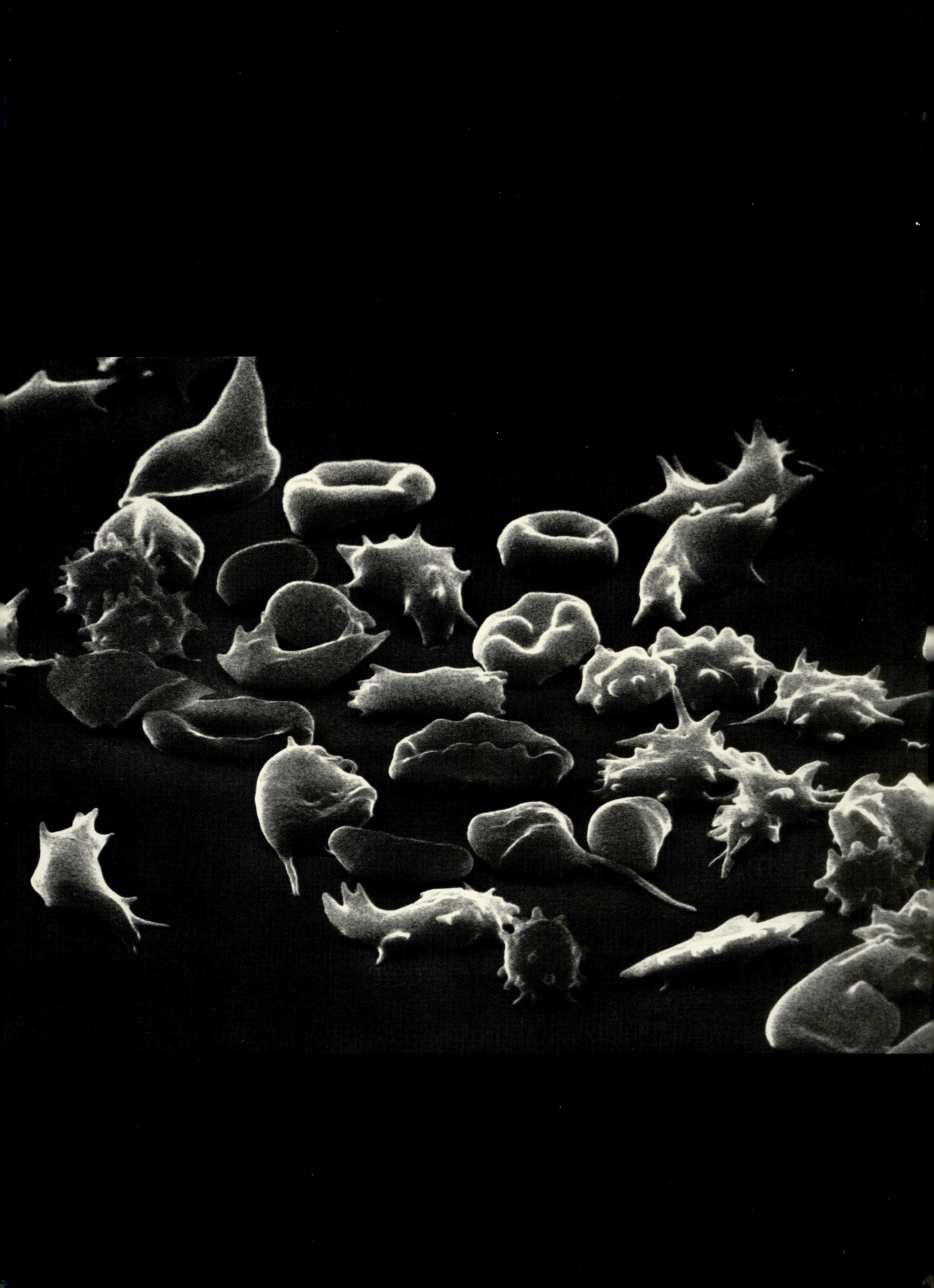

Chapter VII

Keratocytes and Schizocytes

Keratocytes and Schizocytes

Keratocytes are ruptured red cells. Their origin is quite specific. When red cells impinge at high speed on an obstruction, a prosthesis, or a denuded portion of a vessel wall on which intravascular coagulation has taken place, the red cells may be bisected by fibrin strands which adhere to these pathological structures. There is very little loss of hemoglobin in the process. As the red cells are forced against the fibrin strand, virtually all the hemoglobin is pushed into two teardrop- or saddle-shaped portions of the red cell that extend downstream on either side of the strand which holds the cell in place. The opposing interior surfaces of each saddle bag adhere to each other along the fibrin strand so that the hemoglobin is entirely loculated. If eddies in the current tear the entire cell loose from the fibrin attachment, the fused portion of the interior surfaces is now colorless and, in smears, may look like a vacuole. It is usually seen at one edge of the cell. The fused membrane is removed, presumably in the spleen, and the end result is a red cell with two horns, a keratocyte.

At other times the red cell is actually cut, again with a minimal loss of hemoglobin: most of the hemoglobin content of the cell has moved downstream and away from the thin line at which the two saddle bags are still joined. When the cut occurs, the surface reseals instantaneously. The two resulting fragments are often uneven in size and may assume odd shapes such as triangles, rods or crescents. They are referred to as schizocytes.

Keratocytes and schizocytes have been observed especially in so-called micro-angiopathic anemias and after cardiac or vascular surgery.

Keratocytes and schizocytes, like other pathological red cells, can undergo the discocyte-stomatocyte or discocyte-echinocyte transformation and become spheres before hemolysis.

Fig. 1. Keratocyte: a mutilated erythrocyte.

Figs. 2 and 3. Keratocytes. The horn-like structures appear on the edges of the lost portion of the membrane.

Fig. 4. Disco-schizocytes. Red-cell fragments in their discocytic form. *Echino-schizocytes.* Transformation into echinocytic forms occurs in preserved blood.

Fig. 5. Disco-schizocyte and a normal red cell.

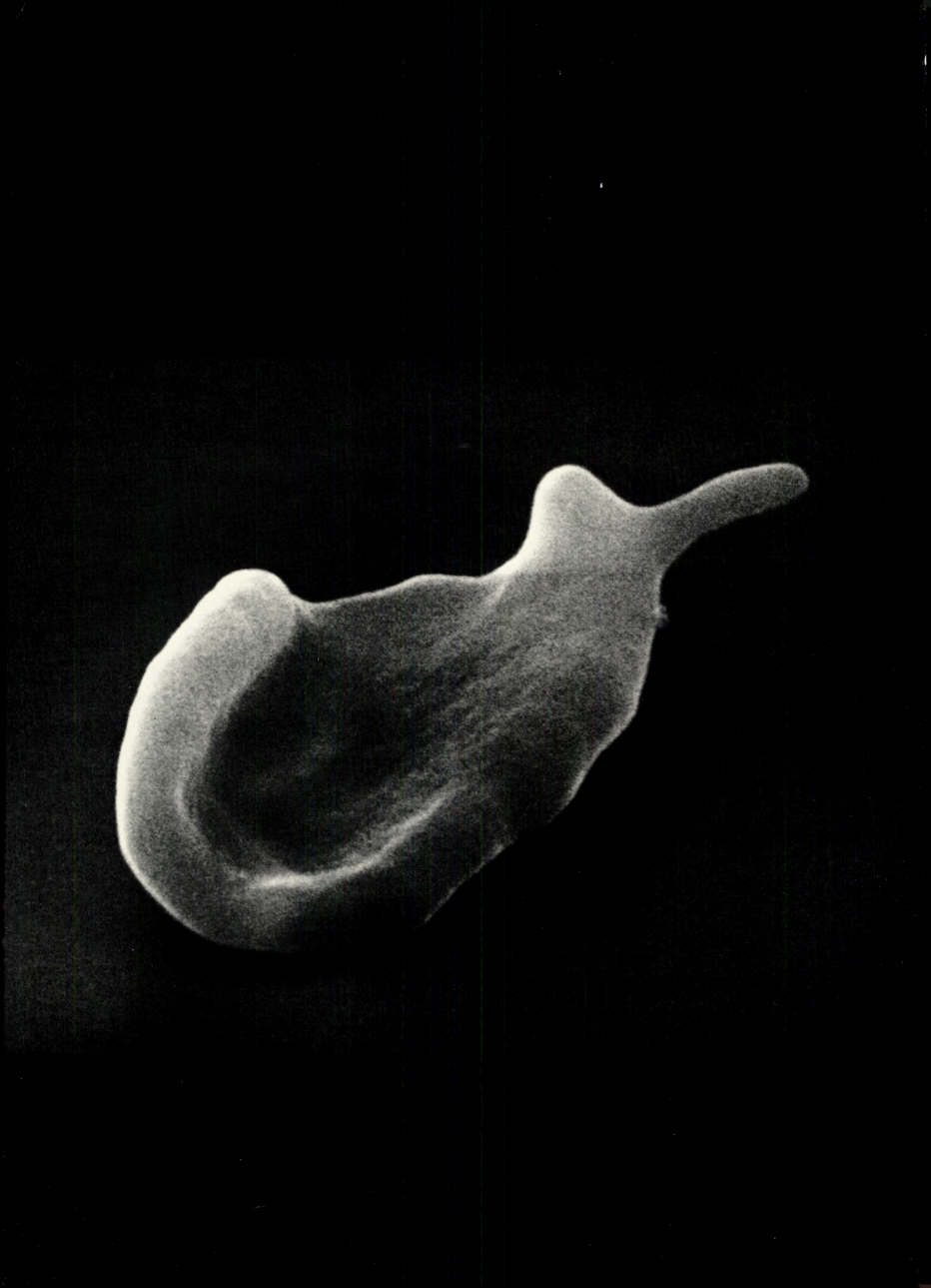

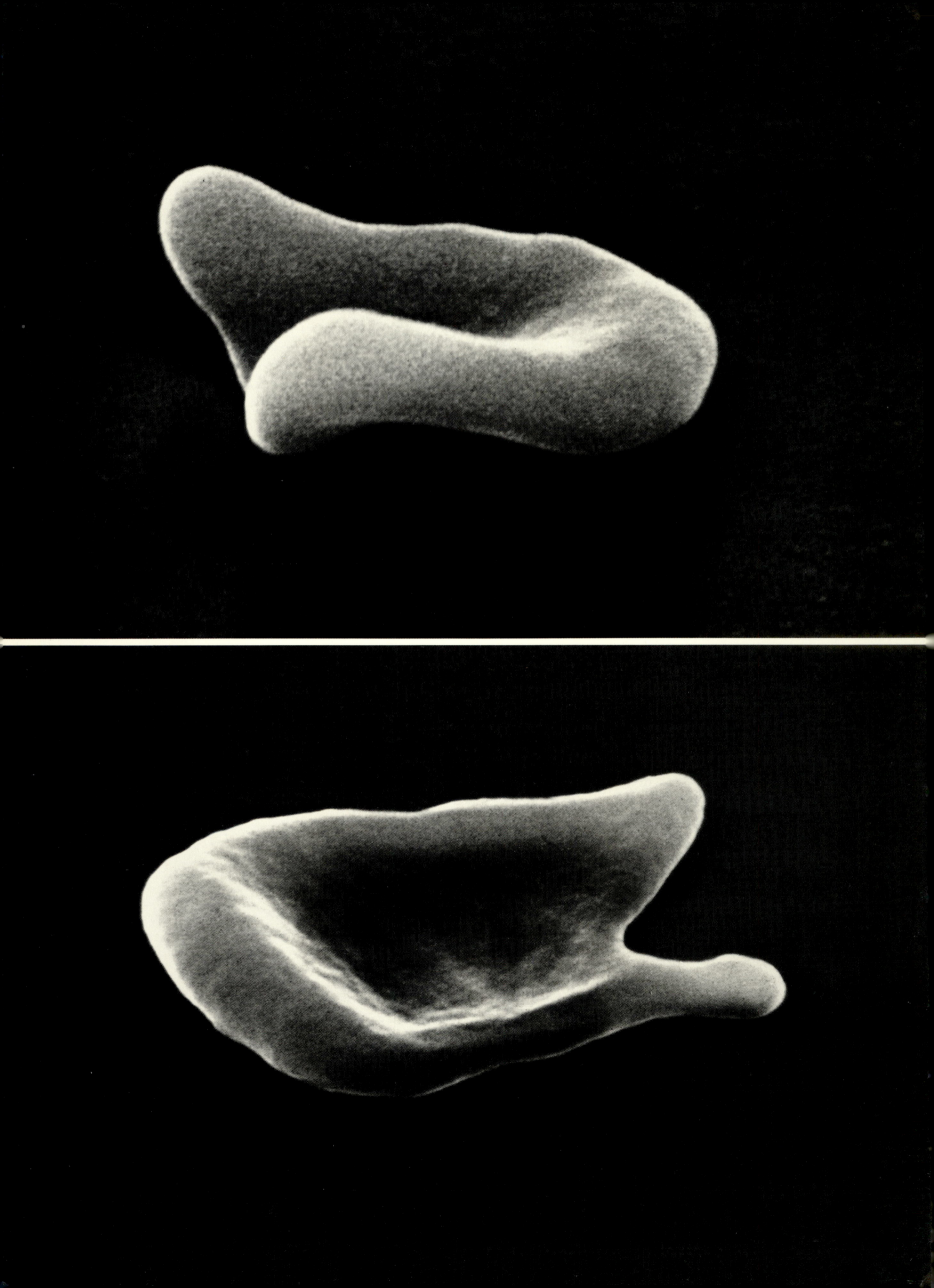

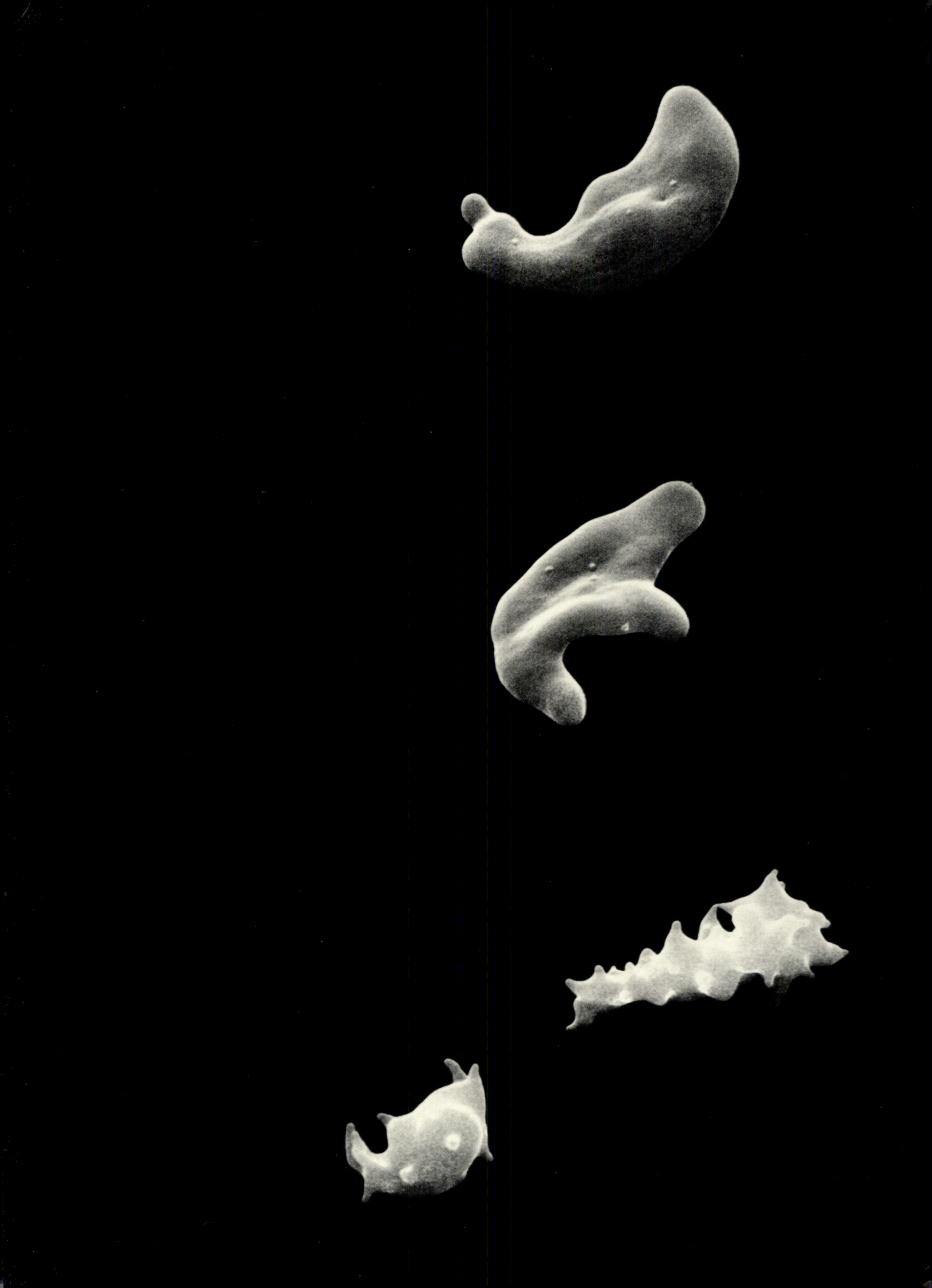

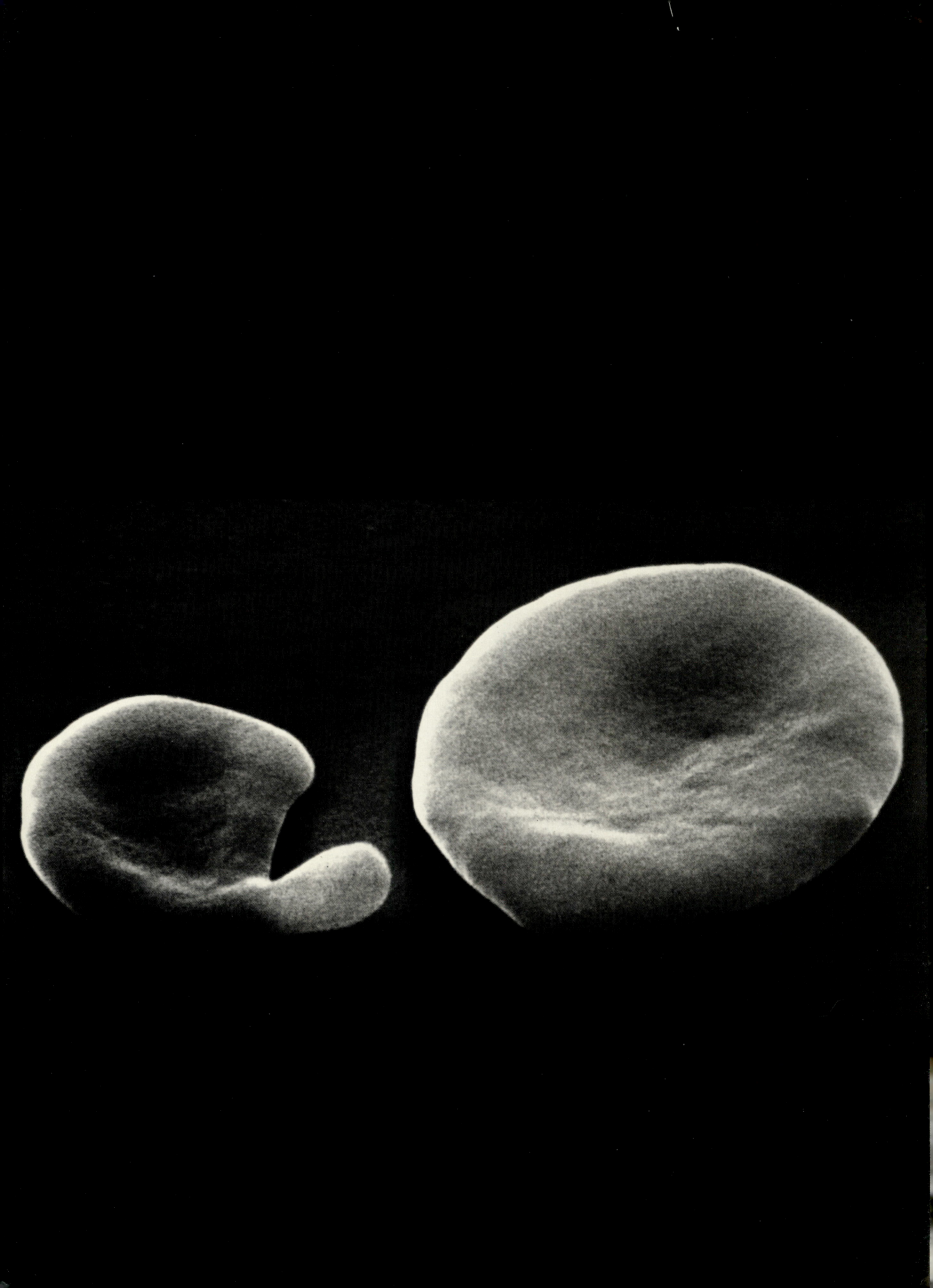

Chapter VIII

Dacryocytes

Dacryocytes

Dacryocyte is the literal translation into Greek of "tear-drop cell," a term which has been in use for a long time. Actually, these cells look more like Chinese porcelain spoons.

The mode of formation of dacryocytes is not completely understood. They are observed in thalassemia, and in leukemic, toxic, and hemolytic anemias.

Like other pathological shapes, dacryocytes can undergo echinocytic and stomatocytic transformation into echino- and stomato-dacryocytes.

Fig. 1. Dacryocyte. This "tear drop" is depressed in its center.

Figs. 2 and 3. Dacryocyte. Comparison between a dacryocyte seen in three dimensions on the right and a similar cell smeared on a glass slide on the left.

Fig. 4. Another dacryocyte. Behind it, a blood platelet.

Figs. 5 and 6. Echino-dacryocytes. Blood from the same patient (thalassemia major) as in the preceding figure, but the preparation has been aged in the incubator for 12 hours. Echino-dacryocytes can be recognized readily.

Fig. 7. Codocyte, dacryocyte, and leptocytes (thalassemia major).

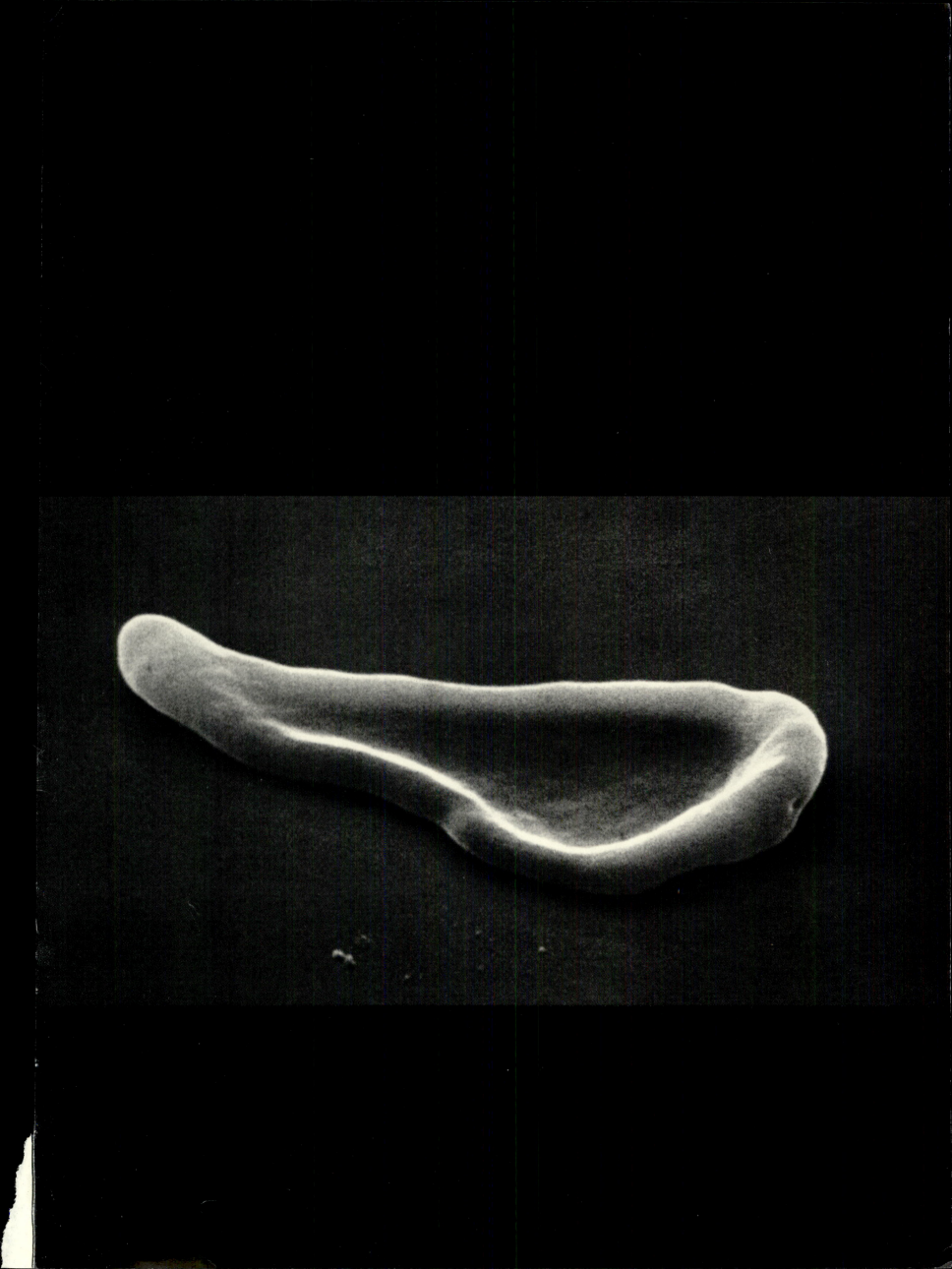

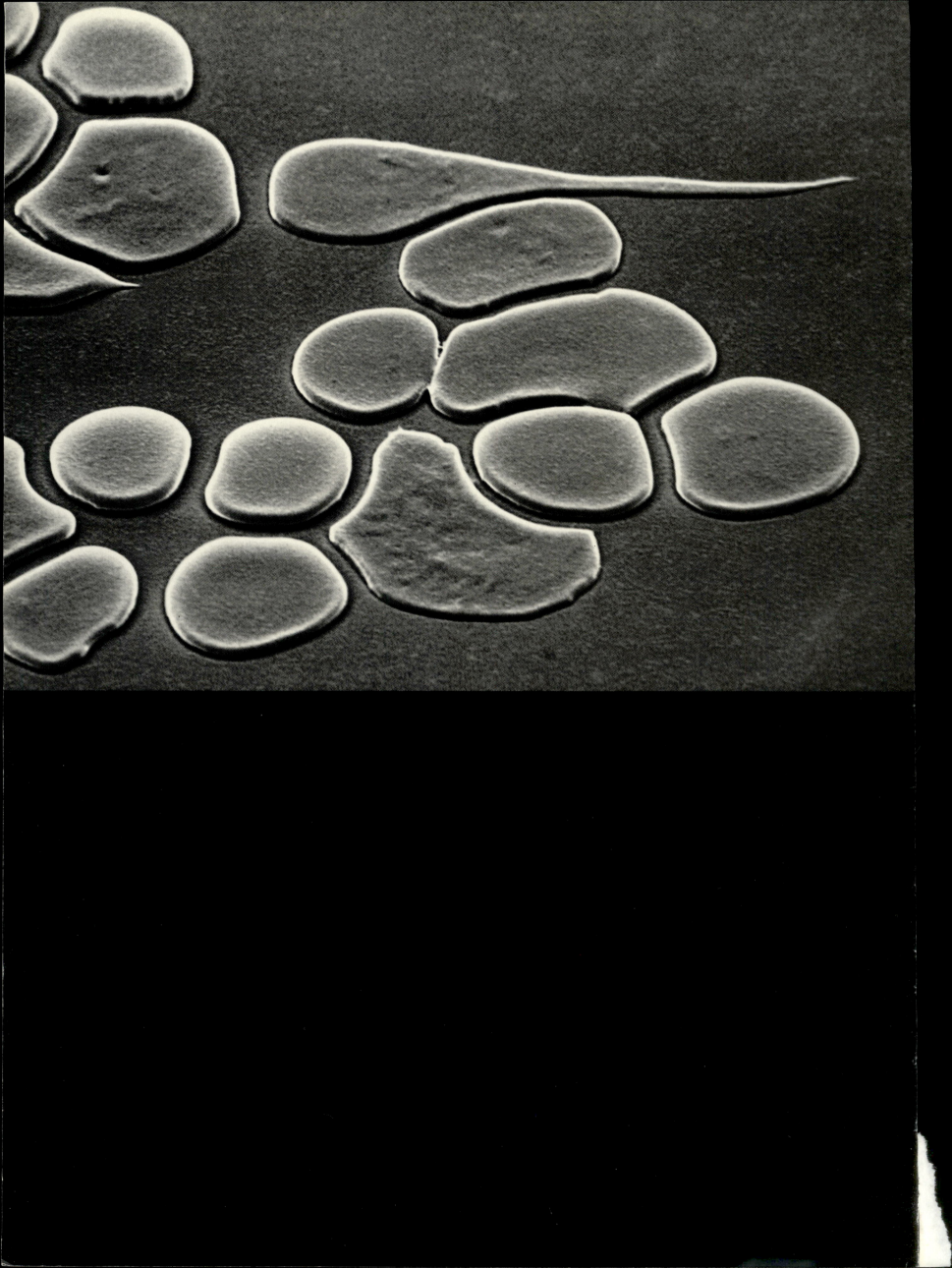

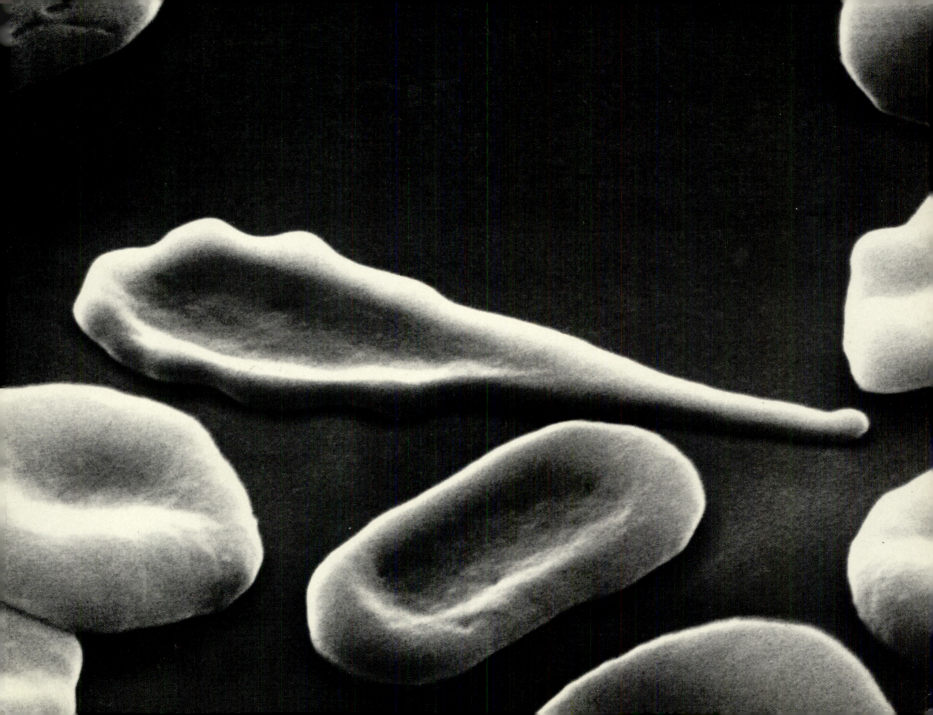

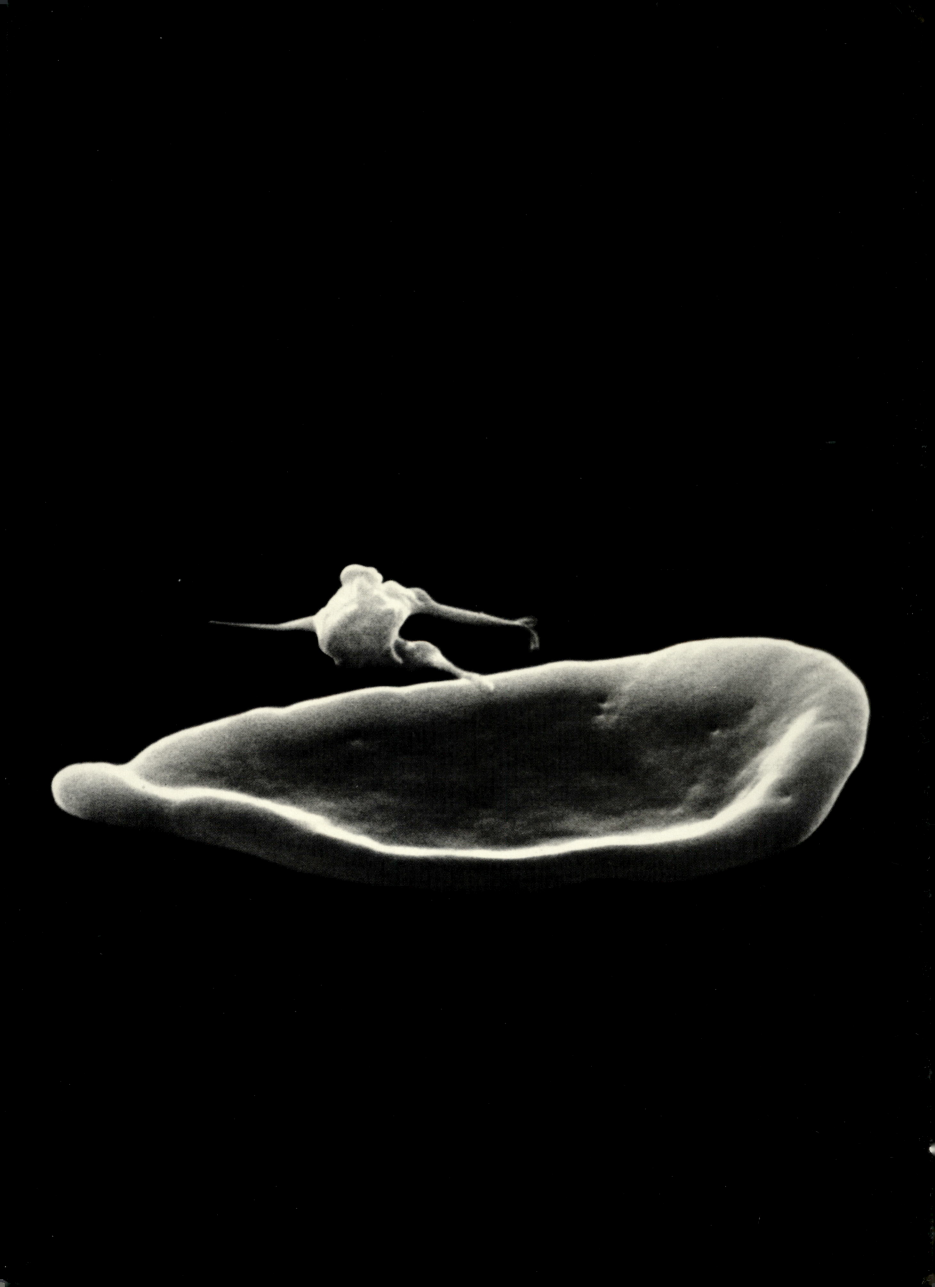

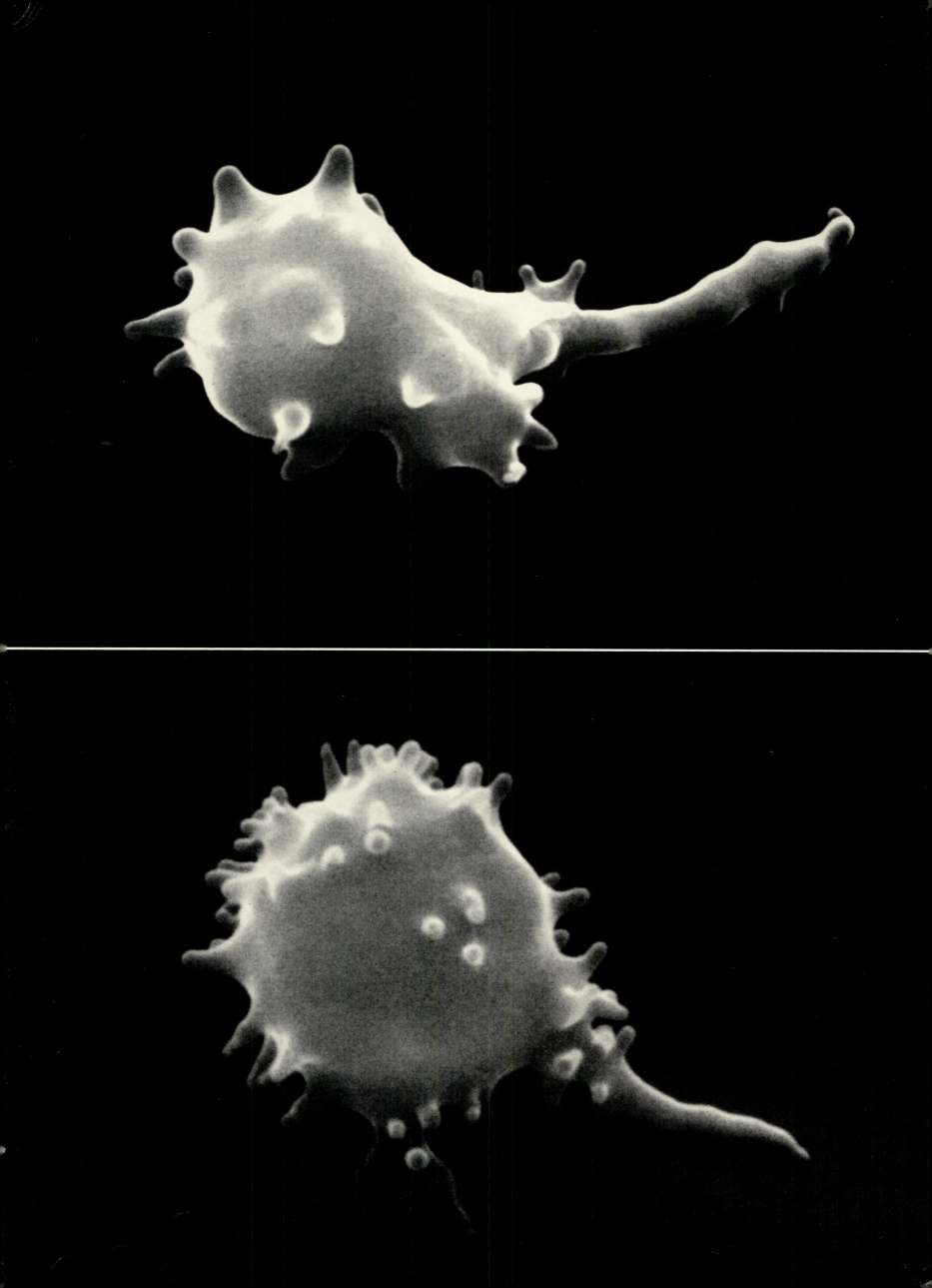

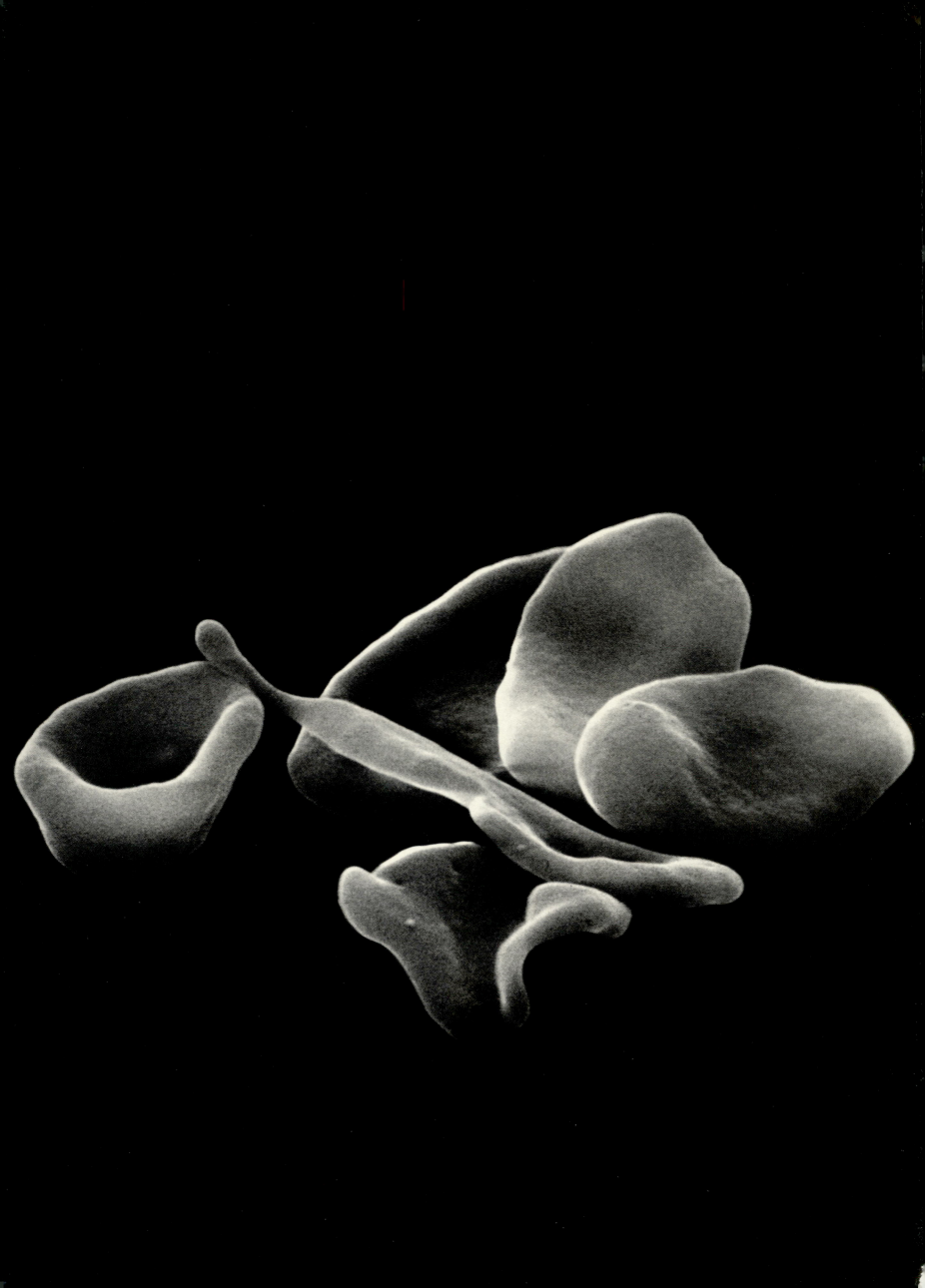

Chapter IX

Codocytes
and
Target Cells

Codocytes and Target Cells

Codocytes are bell-shaped erythrocytes. The "bells" are always thin-walled and should not be mistaken for thick-walled cups or stomatocytes. The mean corpuscular hemoglobin volume and mean corpuscular hemoglobin concentration of codocytes are always low. Codocytes can be thought of as cells whose envelope is too large for their hemoglobin content. Accordingly, their resistance to hypotonic saline is increased, lysis resulting only when the cell membrane is maximally stretched. Codocytes might be considered the antithesis of spherocytes, which have too little membrane for their volume and hence increased susceptibility to lysis or increased "osmotic fragility."

When a smear is prepared and the red cells come to rest flat on the slide, the codocytes with slight concavity will assume the appearance of "target cells."

Target cells (or codocytes) are found in many hypochromic anemias which have a high incidence among persons of Mediterranean or Oriental origin.

Fig. 1. Codocyte I. Hypochromic bell-shaped red cell (Thalassemia).

Fig. 2. Codocyte II. "Mexican-hat" cell.

Fig. 3. Codocyte IV.

Fig. 4. Codocyte IV. Note the small orifice on the concave aspect of the cell. It is probably due to the rupture of a vacuole.

Fig. 5. Codocytes in a smear. Codocytes I and II, with their slight concavity, spread out flat in smears and give the appearance of target cells due to the collapse of their apex; the codocytes III and IV with their deep concavity come to rest on their sides and result in helmet cells.

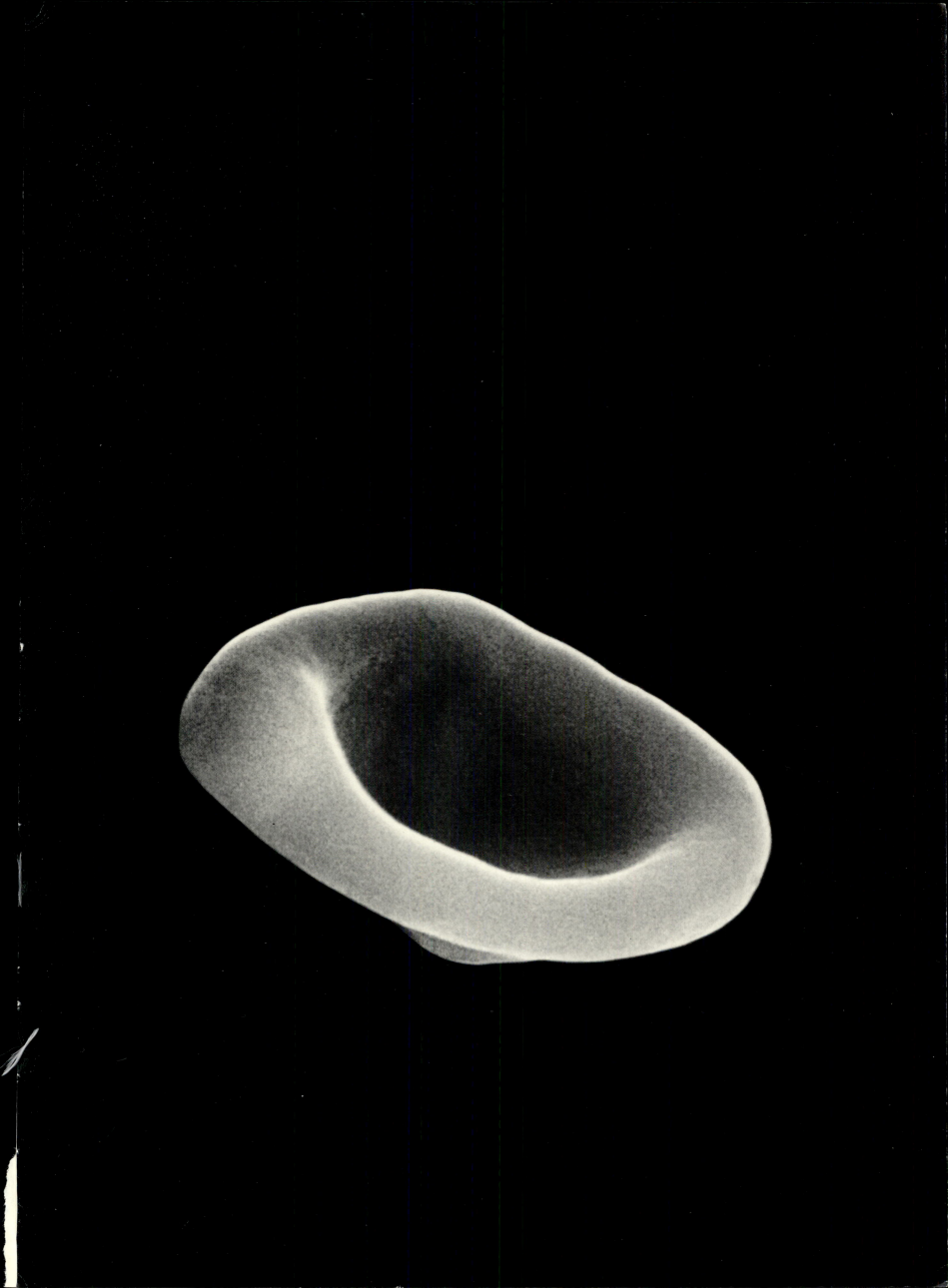

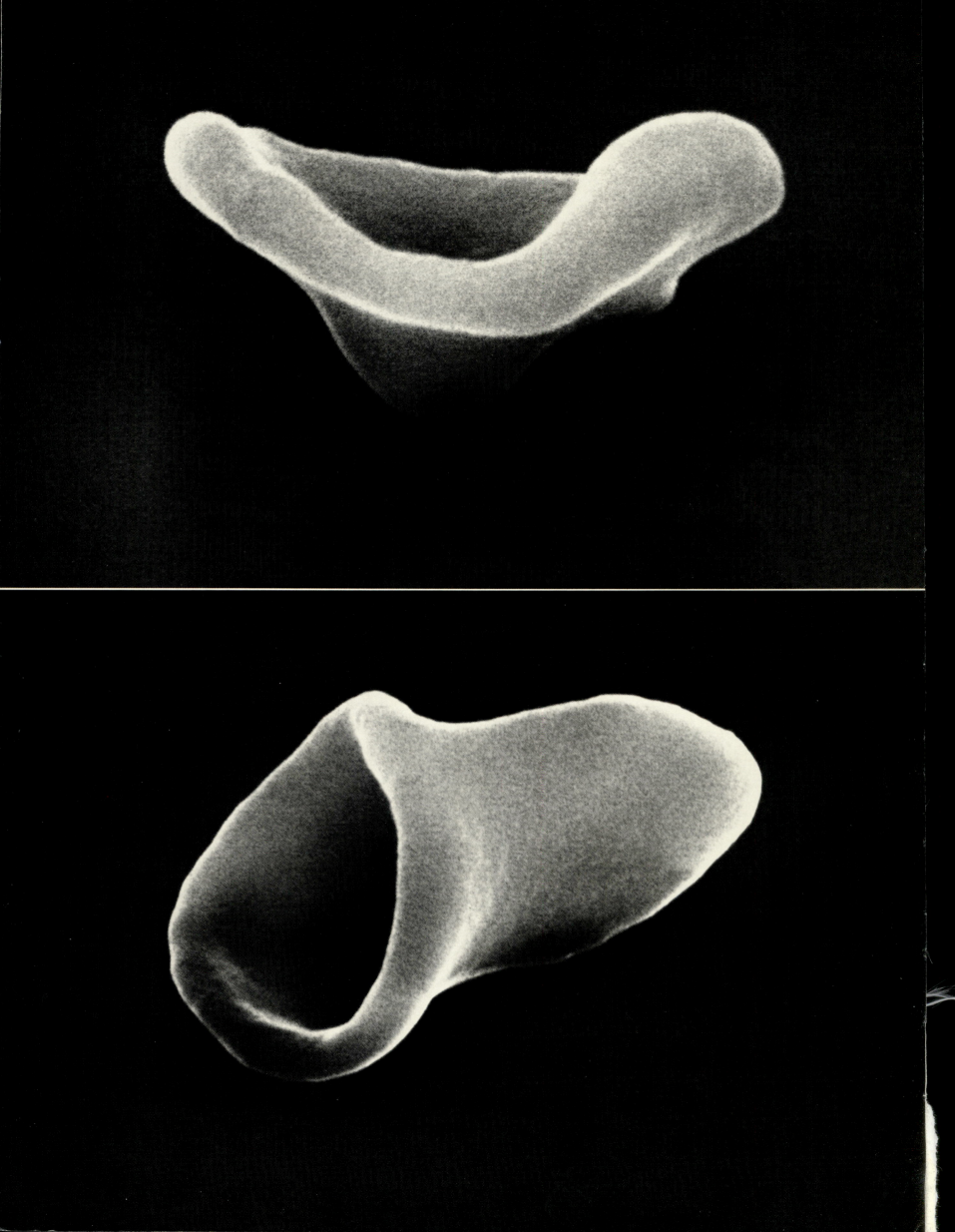

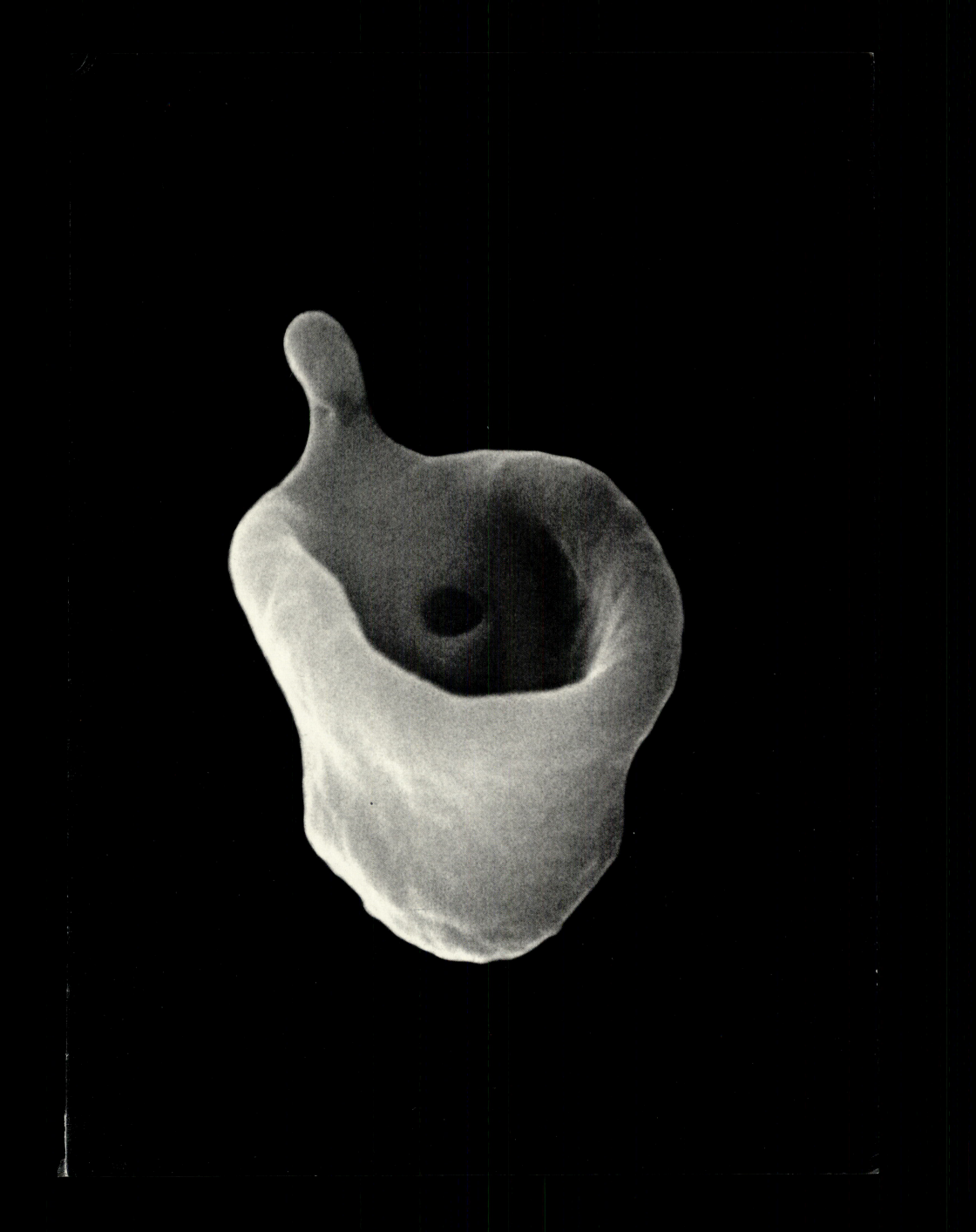

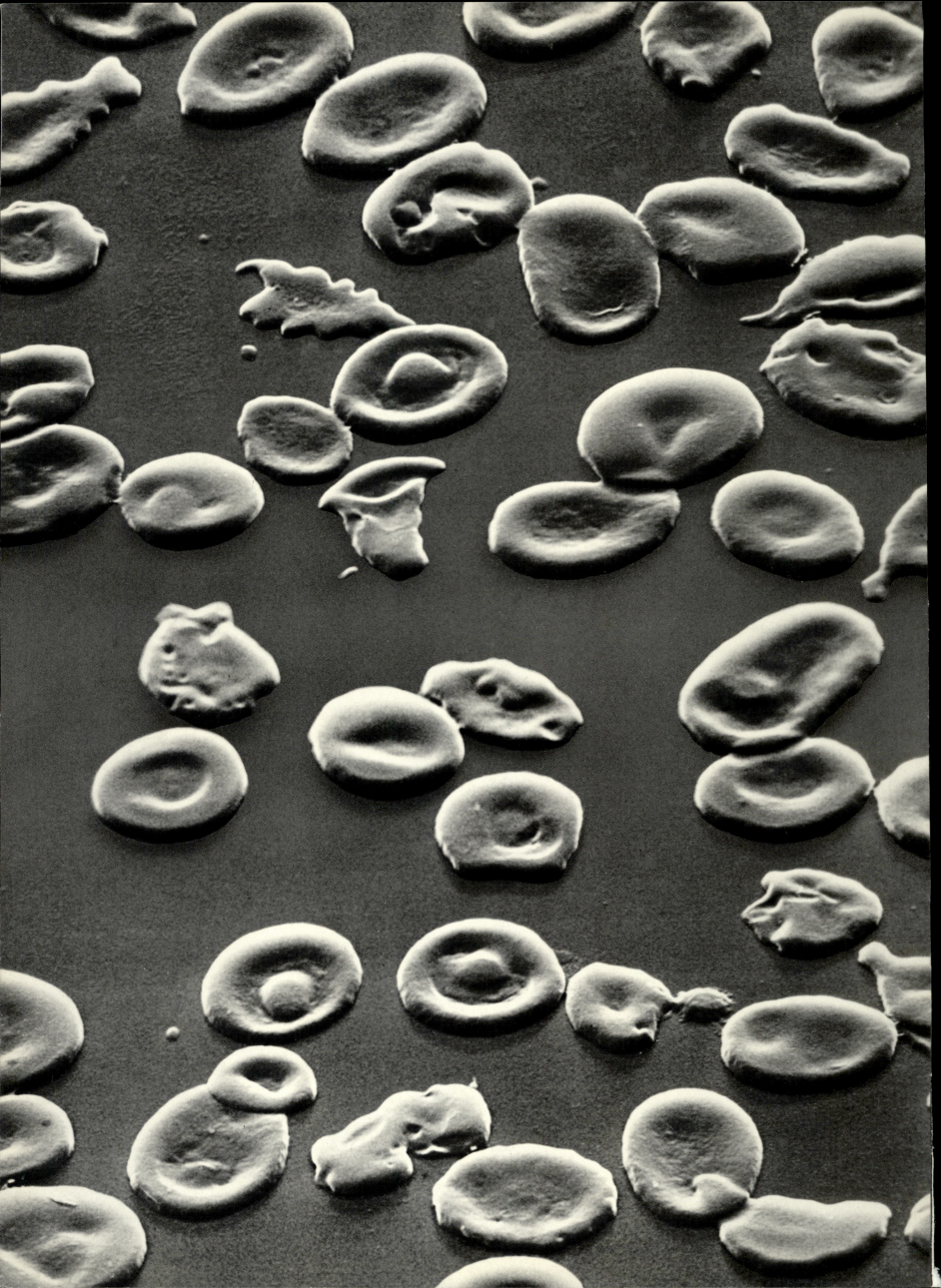

Chapter X

Spherocytes and Knizocytes

Spherocytes

"Spherocytes" is an historical term. The cells it describes are actually not spheres. They include a variety of cells which are etiologically and morphologically dissimilar. They have only one thing in common: an increase in their thickness. At present, we can distinguish: 1. macro-spherocytes produced by osmotic swelling of normal erythrocytes; 2. echino-spherocytes (the extreme form of the disco-echinocyte transformation) and stomato-spherocytes (the extreme form of the disco-stomato-cyte transformation): in these two types of spherocytes the cell volume is normal; 3. micro-spherocytes resulting from fragmentation; 4. the spherocytes seen in hereditary spherocytosis.

Hereditary spherocytosis is a condition in which the red cells tend to be stomato-spherocytes. An allied hereditary condition is hereditary stomatocytosis. The erythrocytes are cup-shaped in the fresh state and present an elongated "mouth" on a smear due to deformation of the cell in the preparation of the smear.

The mechanism of hemolysis in hereditary spherocytosis has been the subject of controversy. Various abnormalities in cell permeability, enzymatic activity and qualitative changes in lipids have been reported. Most of these observations probably reflect secondary phenomena. The underlying defect of the cell membrane has not been identified. It seems clear, however, that the decrease in surface-to-volume ratio involved in sphering makes spherocytes less deformable than discocytes. Sooner or later they are destroyed in the small capillaries and the reticular meshwork of the spleen. Splenectomy thus improves the state of the patient, although the spherocytes persist.

Fig. 1. Spherocyte II. This is in fact a sphero-stomatocyte from a patient with hereditary spherocytosis. In this disease, very few cells are truly spherical. Some have only a minimal central depression, while the majority are stomatocytes II and III. Their diameters appear small but their volume is normal.

Figs. 2, 3, and 4. Progressive alterations in the morphology of a sphero-stomatocyte during the preparation of a smear.

Fig. 5. Stomatocyte I and III.

Fig. 6. Stomatocyte II and knizocyte.

Fig. 7. Knizocytes are triconcave erythrocytes. They can be seen in hereditary or other spherocytoses. They can also be produced by experimental manipulations or occur as artifacts of desiccation during preparation of normal red cells for scanning electron microscopy.

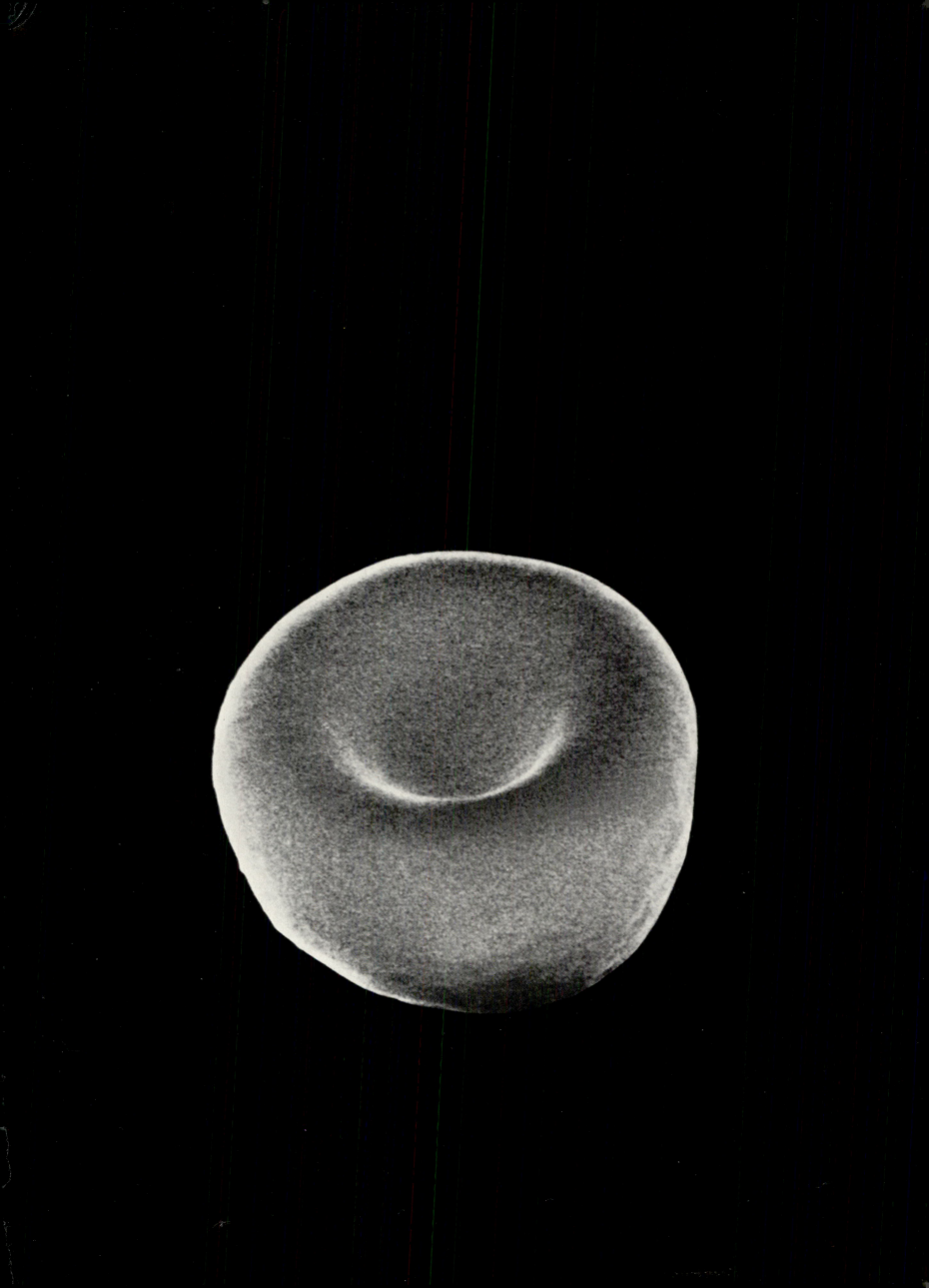

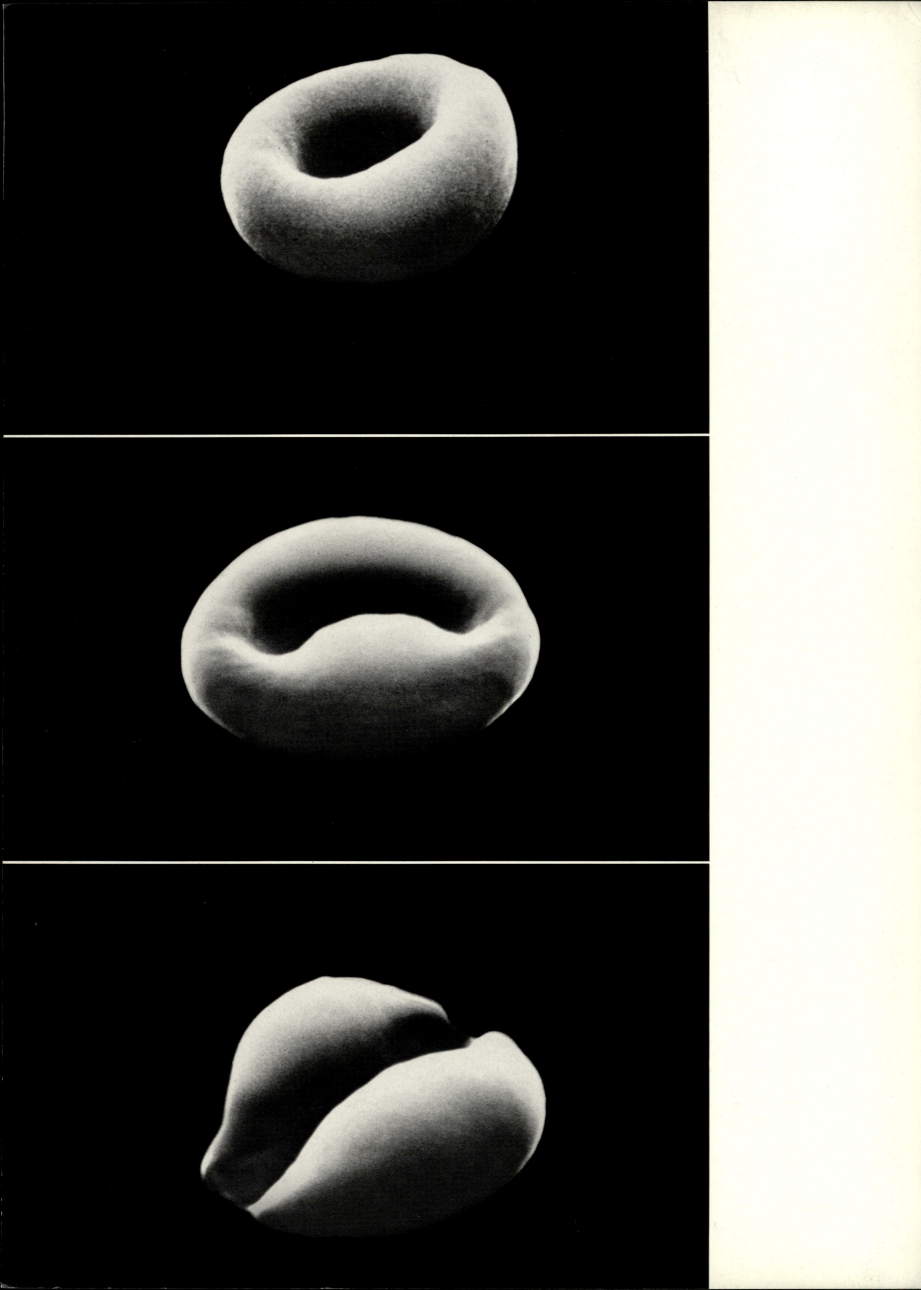

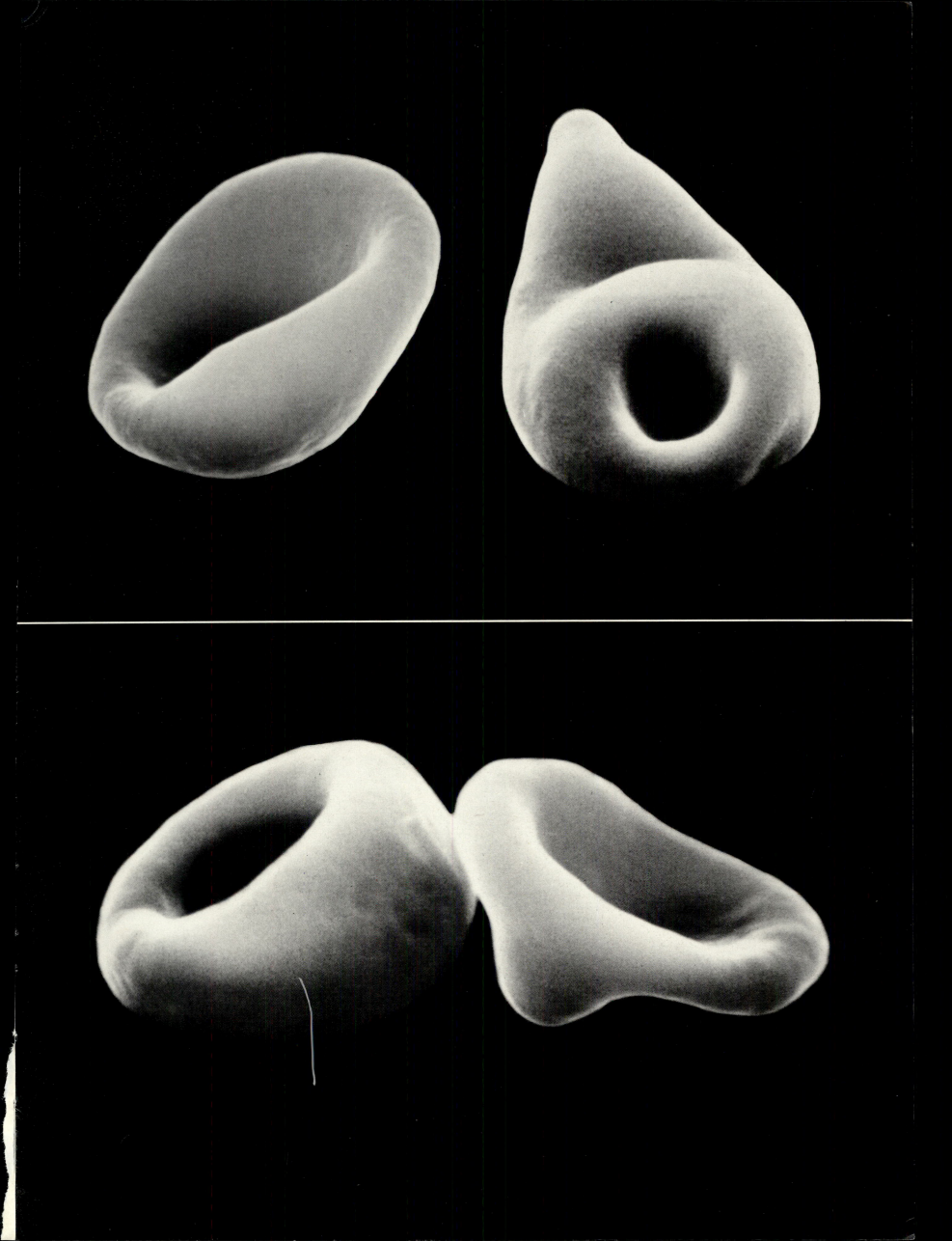

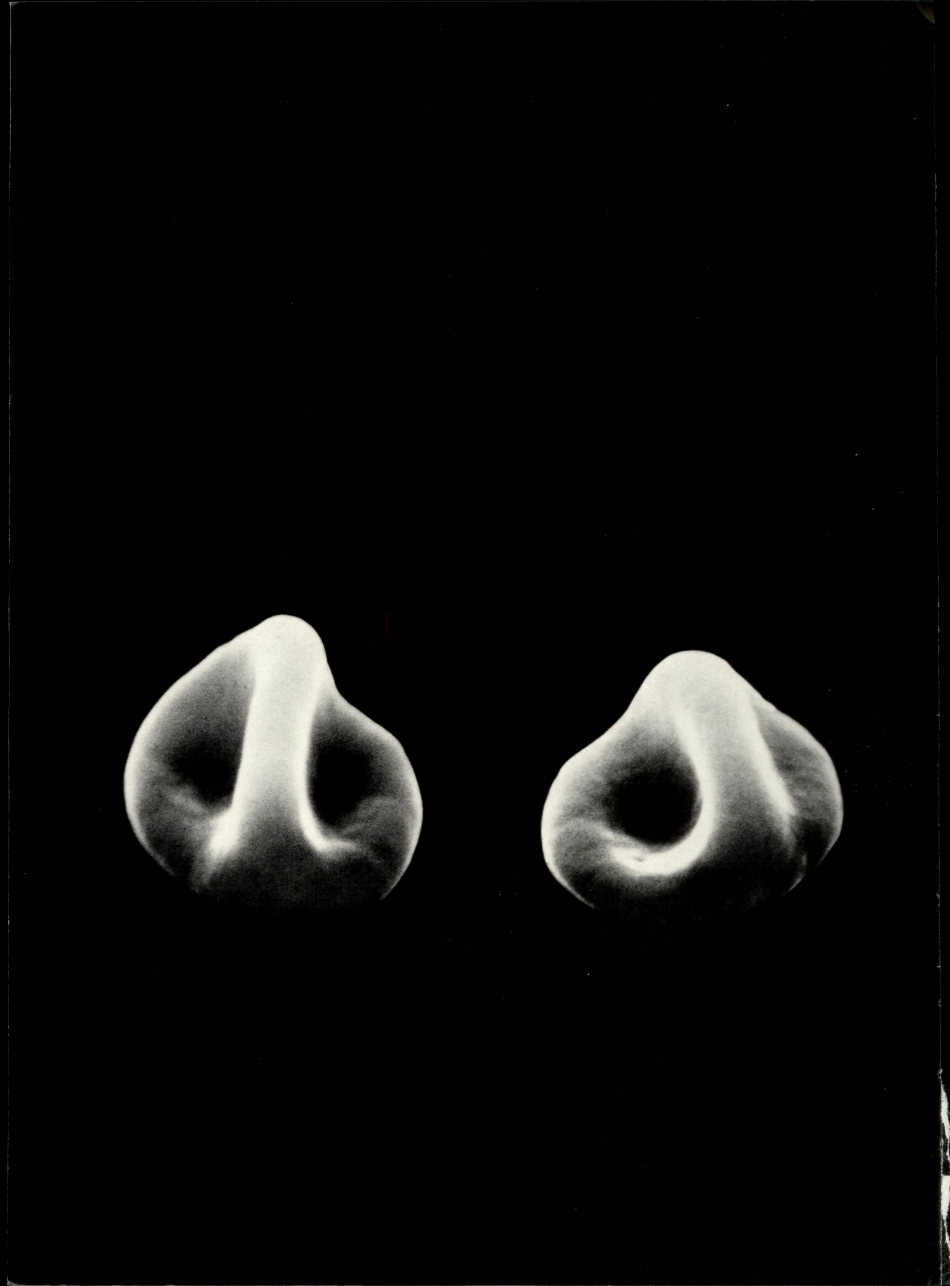

Chapter XI

Elliptocytes

Elliptocytes

Elliptical red cells occur in many anemias. The degree of deviation from the circular shape of discocytes varies from cell to cell in acquired anemias and often only a few elliptocytes are seen. In hereditary elliptocytosis virtually all cells are elliptocytes. Hereditary elliptocytes may or may not be associated with pathological symptoms (hemolysis).

Various classifications of elliptical cells based on the length-to-width ratio have been suggested. For example, one might designate nearly circular cells as group I, oval cells group II, elongated ones group III, and bacilliform ones group IV.

Elliptocytes in man are slightly biconcave. They resemble the oval cells of camels, but human elliptocytes have no increased resistance to osmotic hemolysis as camel cells do. In the desert, camels lose up to one-third of their weight, after which they are capable of drinking up to 130 liters of water in 10 minutes. In man, absorption of 6 liters of water is enough to bring about osmotic hemolysis.

Fig. 1. Elliptocyte II (Hereditary Elliptocytosis).

Figs. 2 and 3. Elliptocytes II.

Fig. 4. Elliptocyte III.

Fig. 5. Echino II-elliptocyte II. This shape is obtained by aging of disco-elliptocytes.

Fig. 6. Sphero-echino I-elliptocyte III.

Fig. 7. Sphero-echino II-elliptocyte III.

Figs. 8 and 9. Echino III-elliptocyte II.

Fig. 10. Stomato II-elliptocyte III. This shape is obtained by the action of chloropromazine on disco-elliptocytes.

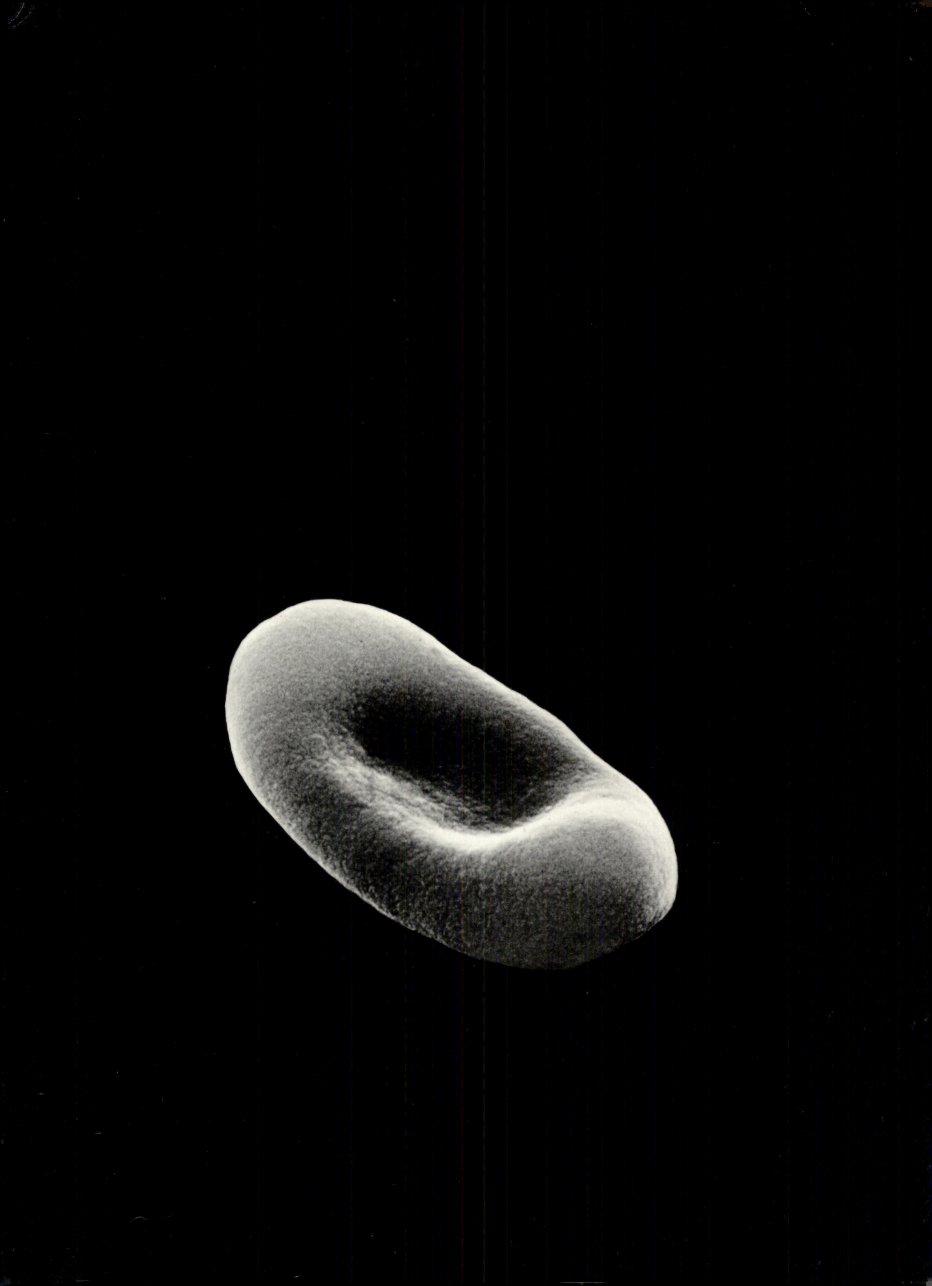

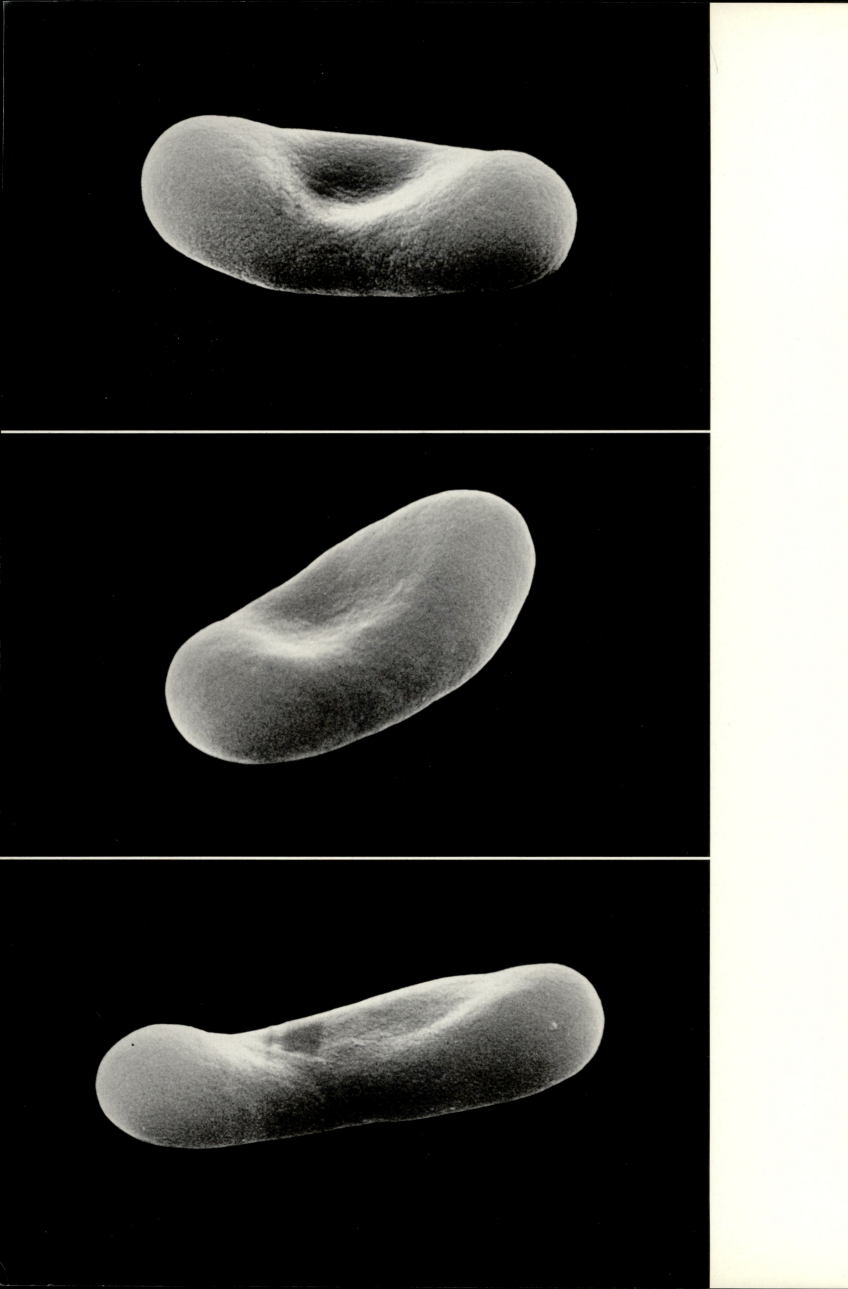

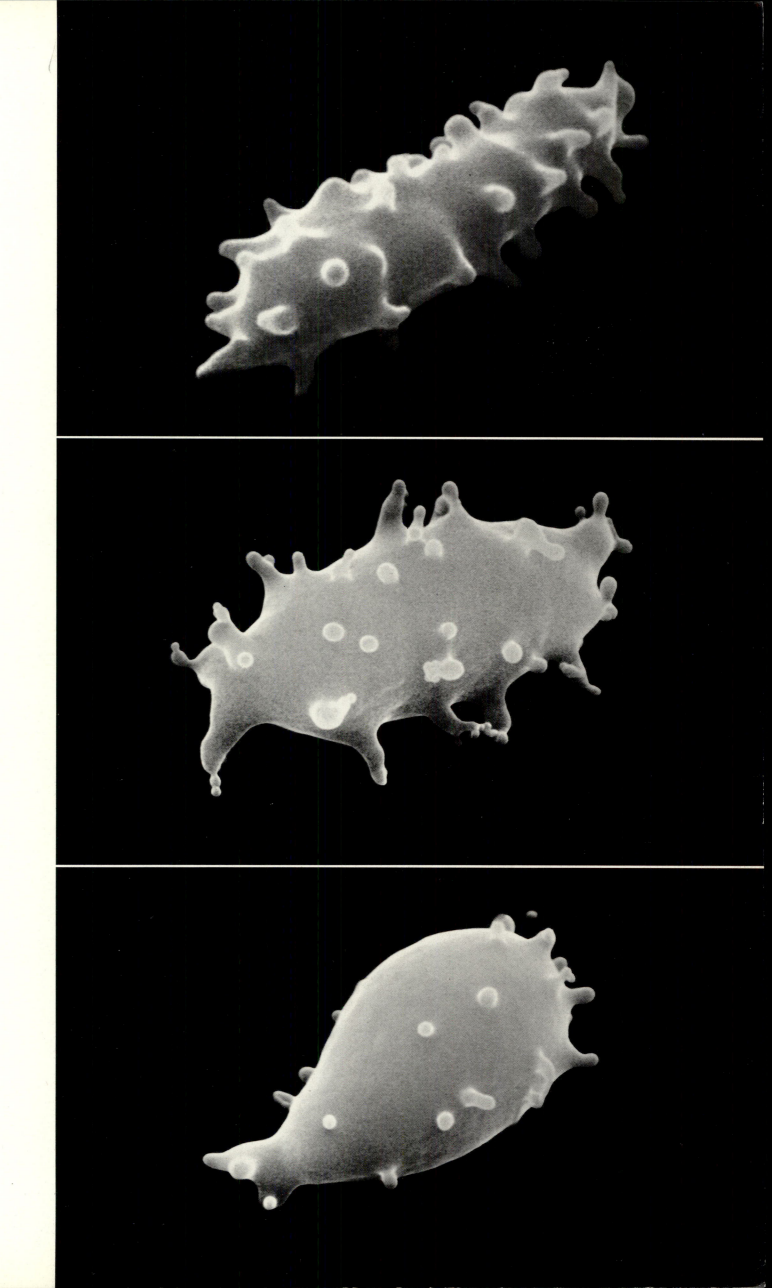

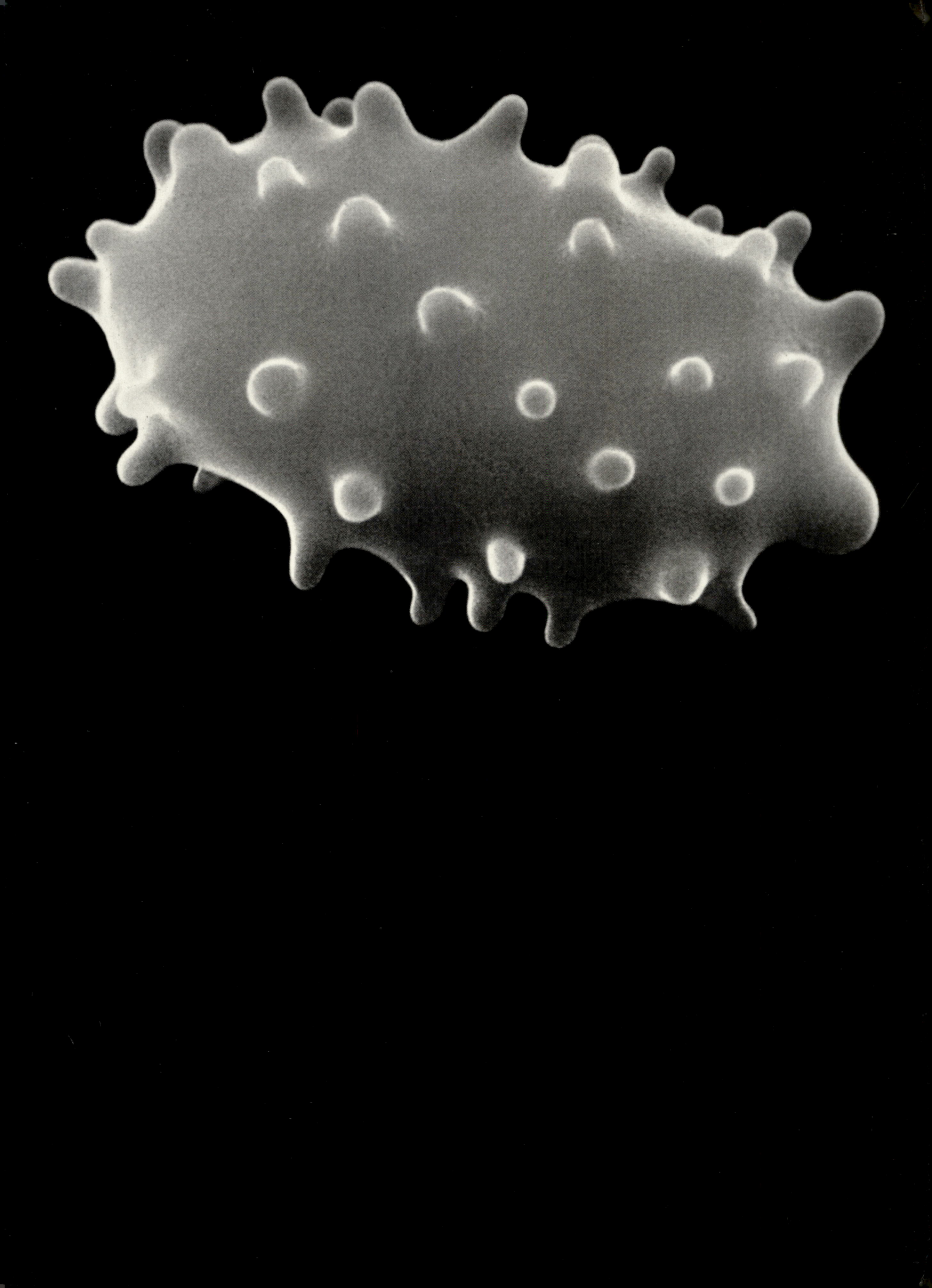

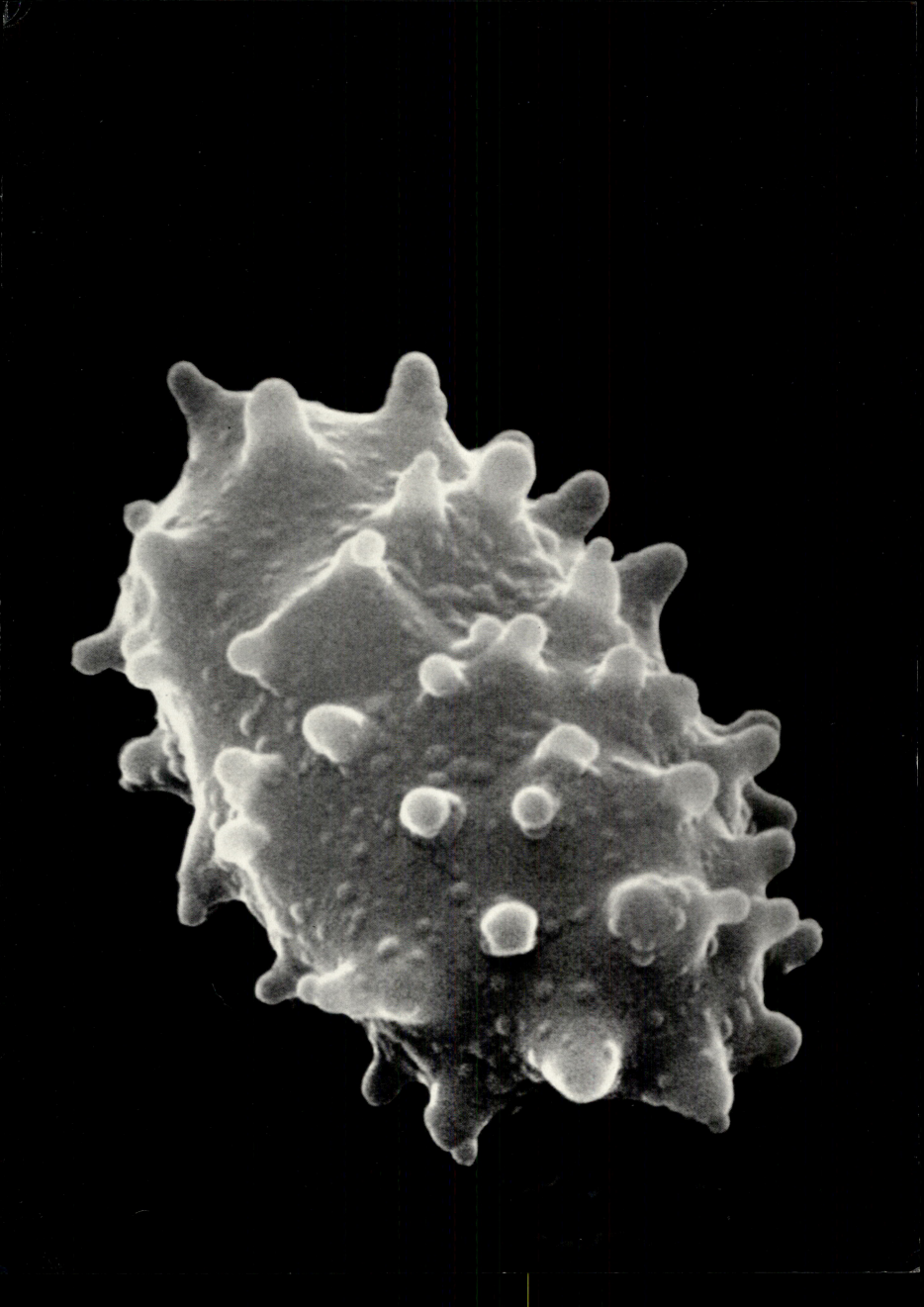

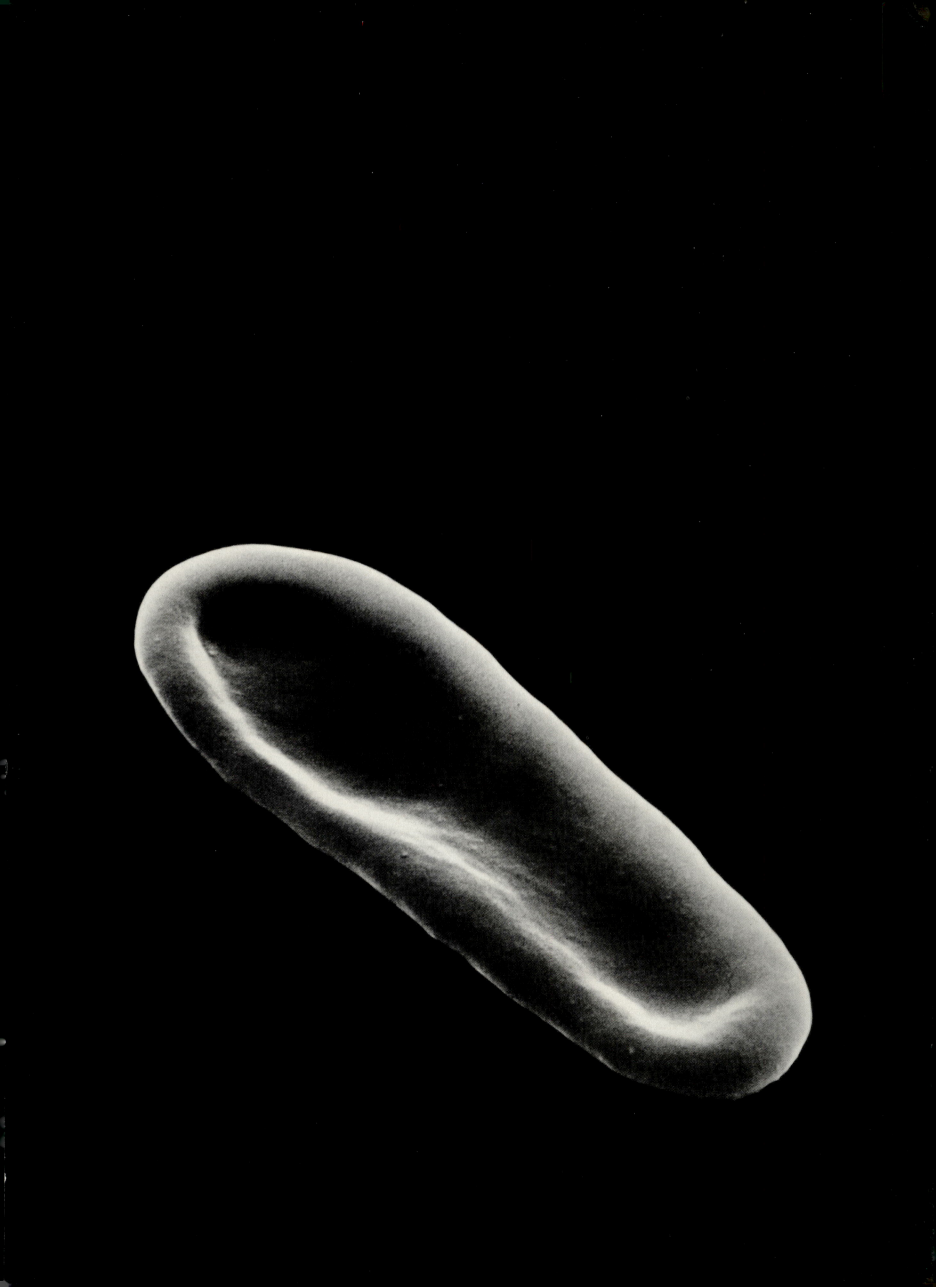

Chapter XII

Acanthocytes

Acanthocytes

Acanthocytes are a very peculiar form of spiculated red cells found in a rare hereditary disease characterized by the absence of beta-lipoprotein (acanthocytosis), in certain cirrhoses of the liver associated with hemolytic anemia, and in rare cases of hepatitis.

Scanning electron microscopy reveals that acanthocytes have very characteristic shapes and that they bear only a superficial resemblance to echinocytes. They have far fewer spicules, and the spicules are irregularly arranged and have knobby ends. Furthermore, acanthocytes are not reversible to discocytes when washed in normal plasma. The plasma of these patients retains the capacity of normal plasma to revert echinocytes to discocytes.

When one exposes acanthocytes to echinogenic factors, new spicules appear, superimposed on the primary spicules, and the acanthocytes become echino-acanthocytes. When acanthocytes are treated with stomatogenic agents, they develop a central concavity. As further stomatocytic change is progressively superimposed on the acanthocyte, its spicules tend to disappear until the cell is completely transformed into a cup-shaped form.

Fig. 1. Acanthocyte III.

Figs. 2 and 3. Acanthocytes III.

Figs. 4 and 5. Echino-acanthocytes, produced by aging of the blood. Note the appearance of finer spicules superimposed on the primary spicules.

Figs. 6, 7, and 8. Stomato-acanthocytes, produced by exposing the cells to low pH or phenothiazine. In Fig. 8, all but one of the spicules have been effaced by the development of the sphero-stomatocytic form.

Fig. 9. Acanthocyte I.

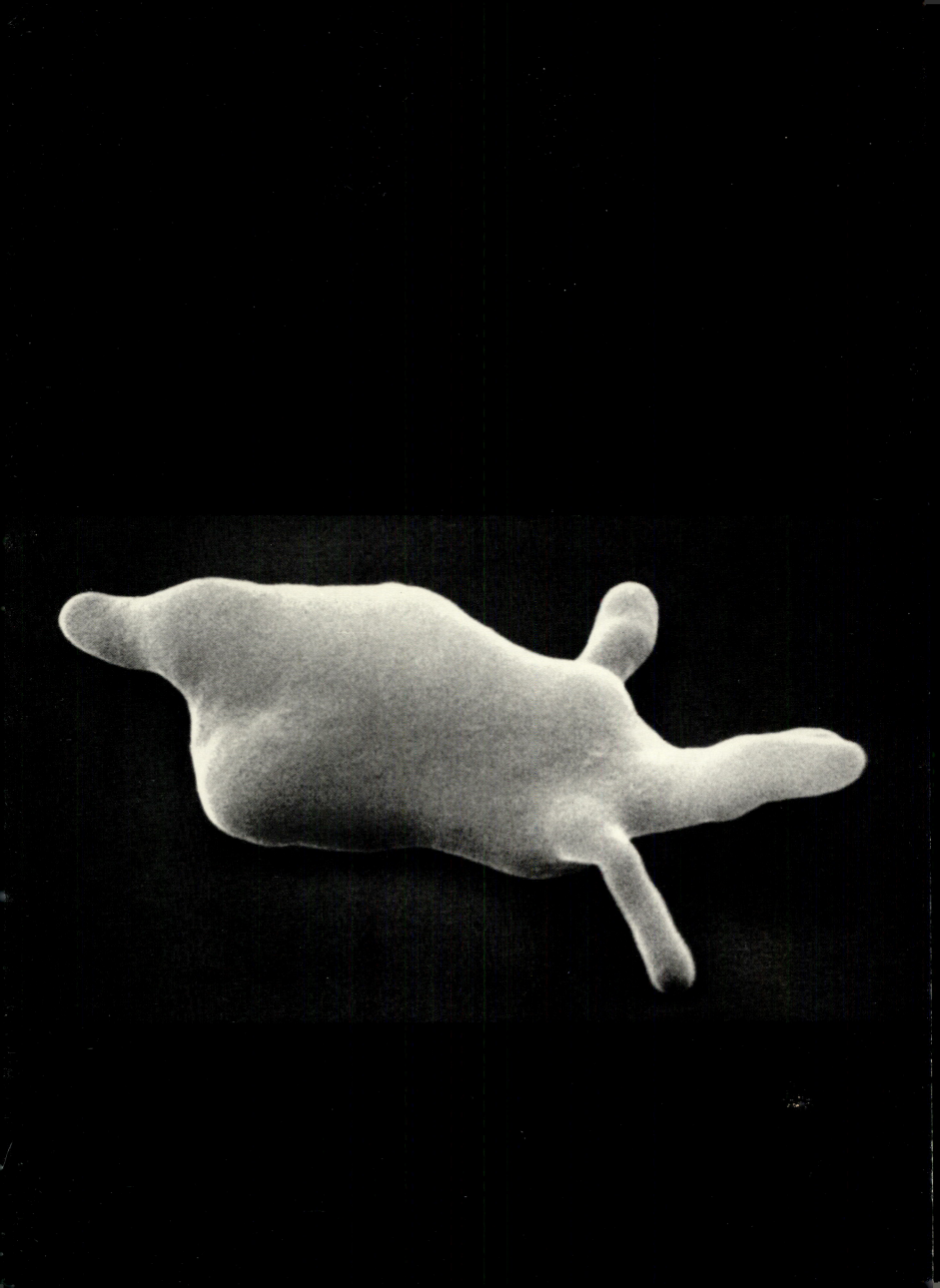

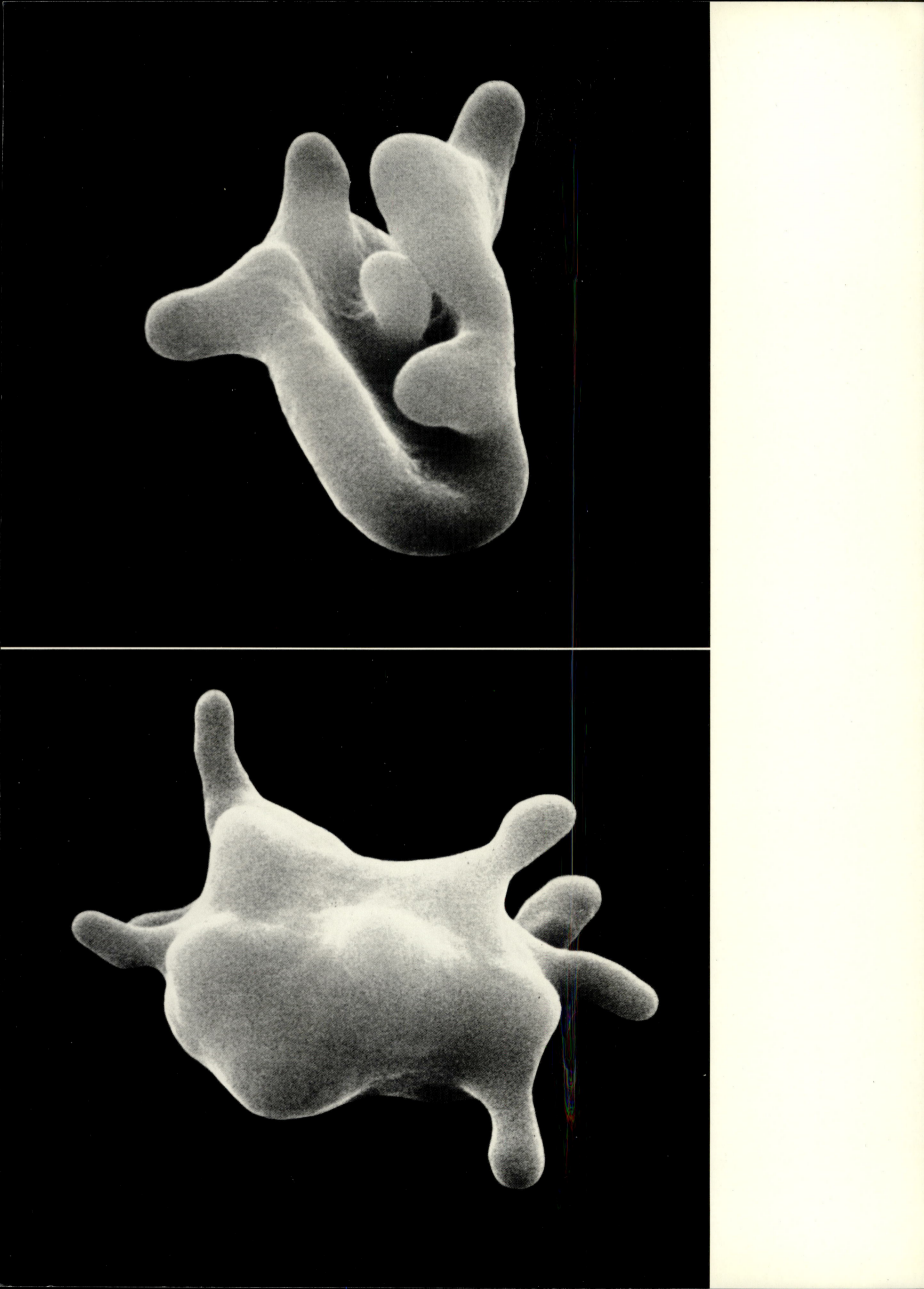

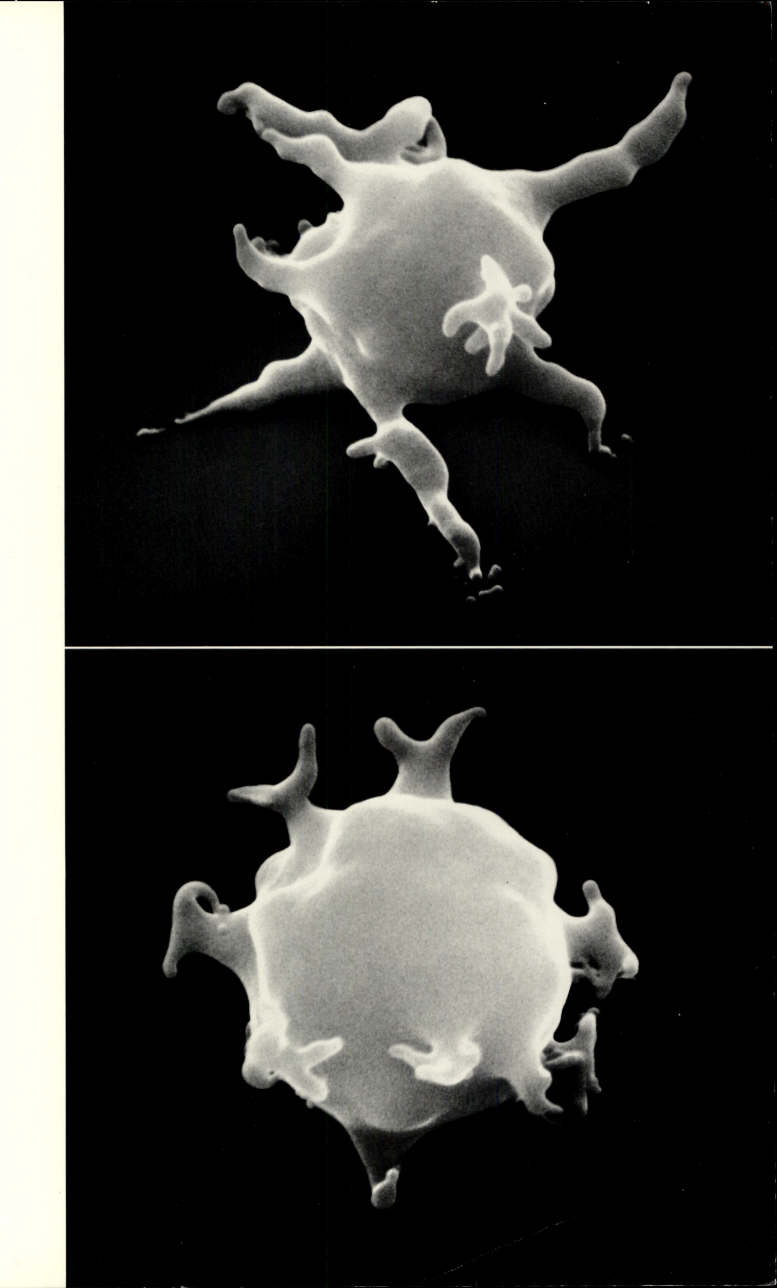

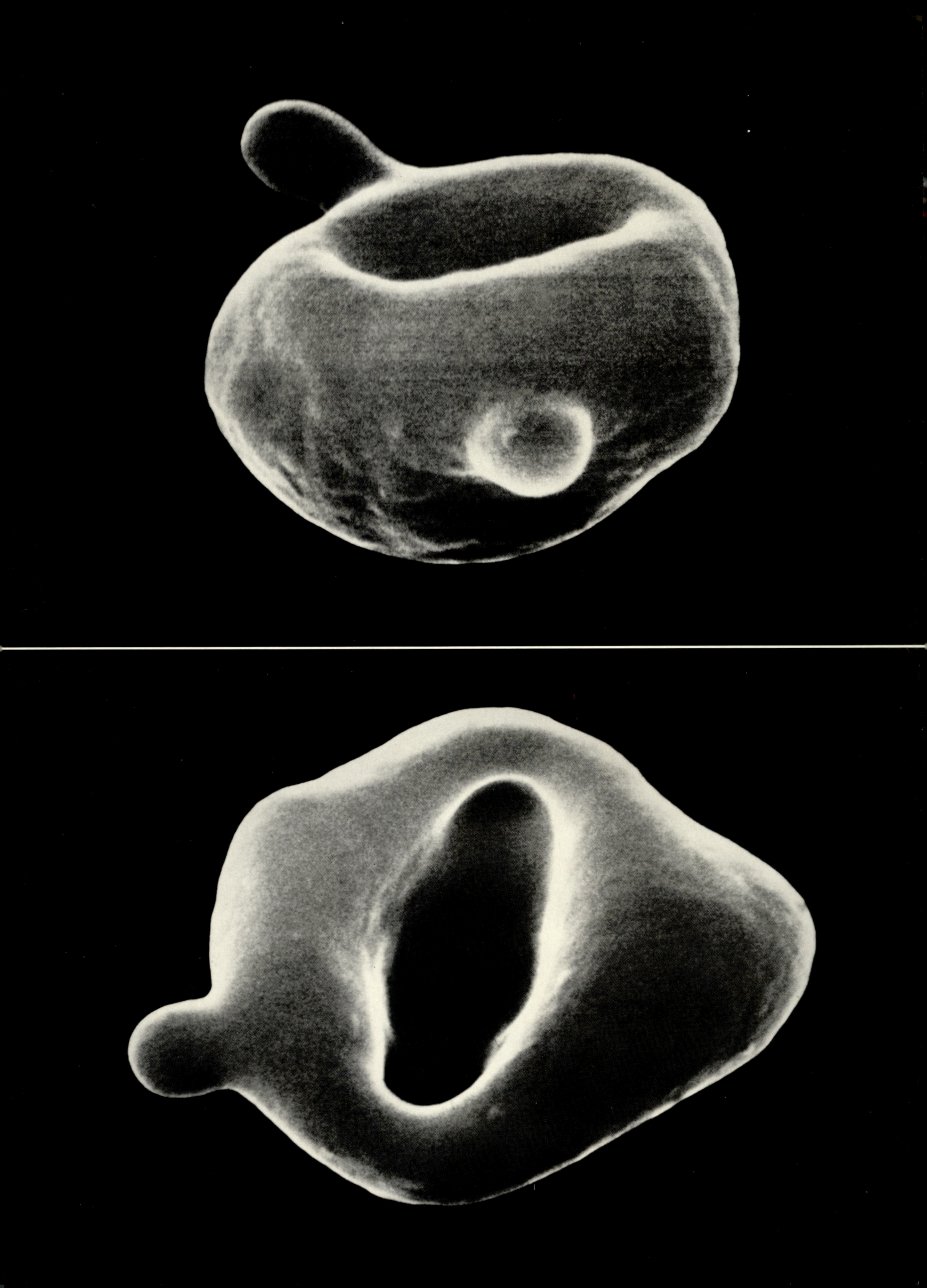

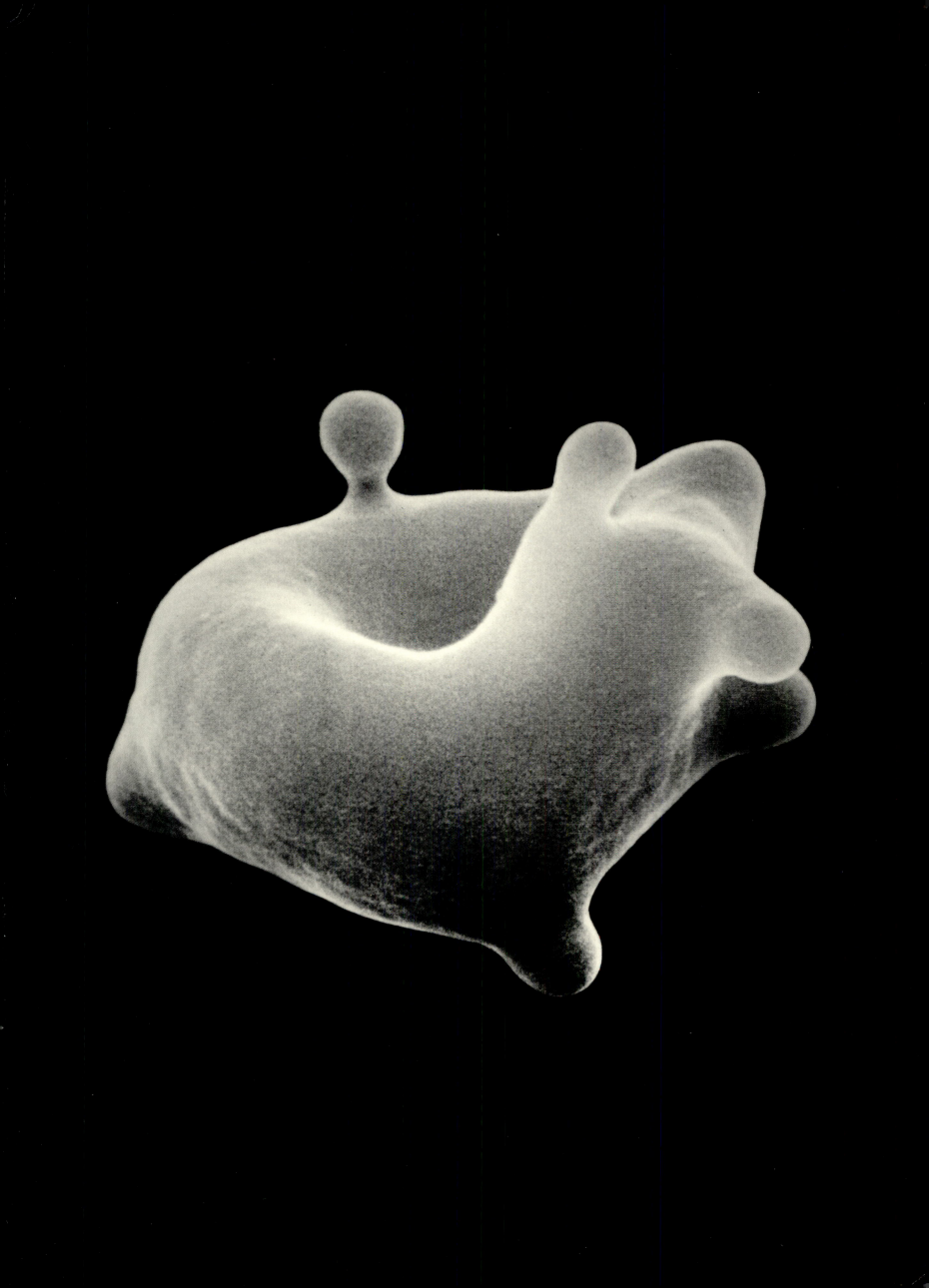

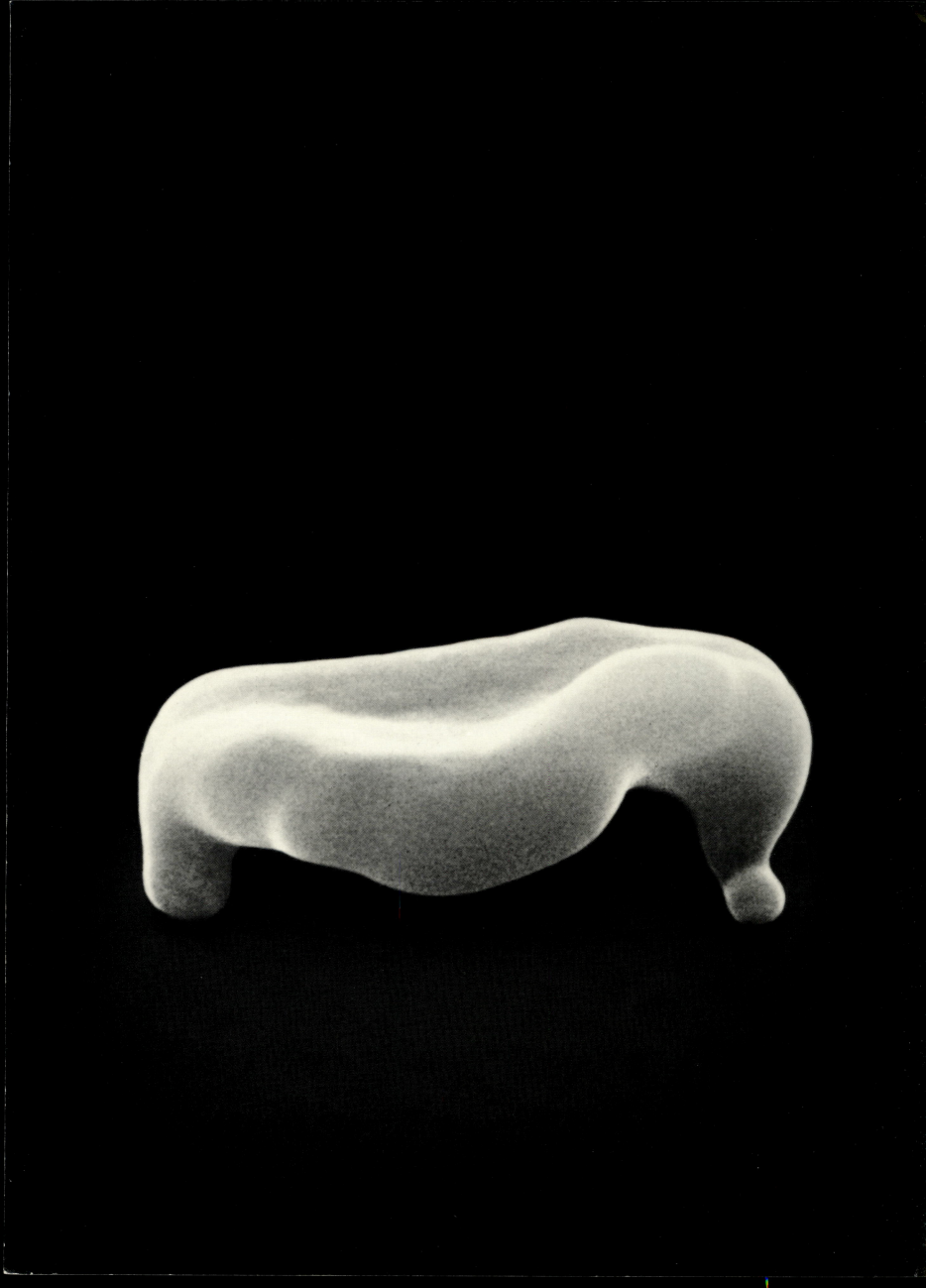

Chapter XIII

Zoo

Zoo

This chapter is irrelevant—like the thirteenth floor in good hotels, it should be regarded as non-existent. Perhaps, none-theless, some frivolous minds will enjoy this peculiar photo-graphic safari, and recognize some of the game: acanthocytes, keratocytes, schizocytes and other target cells . . .

Description of Plates

1   *Uburex Filamentosus* (Jarr.), exhibiting its antenna.
2   *Garabagnus Nobilis* (Michau.).
3   *Garabagnus Nobilis* (Michau.), female, on its back.
4   *Scarabeus Ferox* (Kafk.).
5   *Uburex Filamentosus* (Jarr.), standing up.
6   *Limacca Rubesca* (Coust.).
7   *Microcerotus Sanguinotulus* (Ionesc.).
8   *Potheas Amphibius* (Bosch.).
9   *Flamina Flammea* (Fredou.).
10   *Capucinus Gutturalis Mandonii* (Bosch.).
11   *Maco-Mokiki Alycius* (Carrol.).
12   *Echinoptera Hirta* (Coust.) and *Limacca Rubra* (Coust.).
13   *Disconidus Fuliginosus* (Coust.).
14   *Echinoptera Hirta* (Coust.) and *Faustina Juanica* (Miro.).

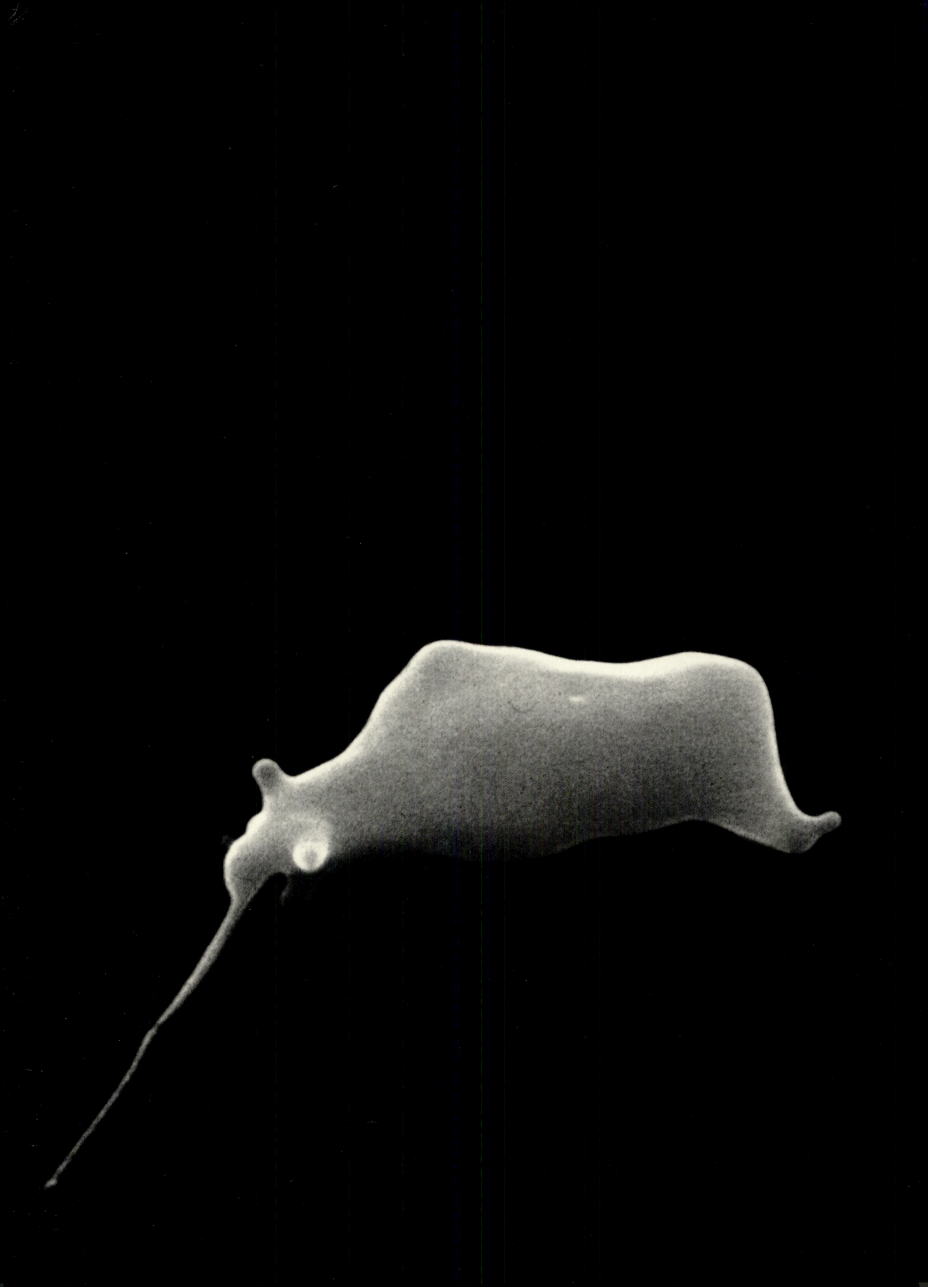

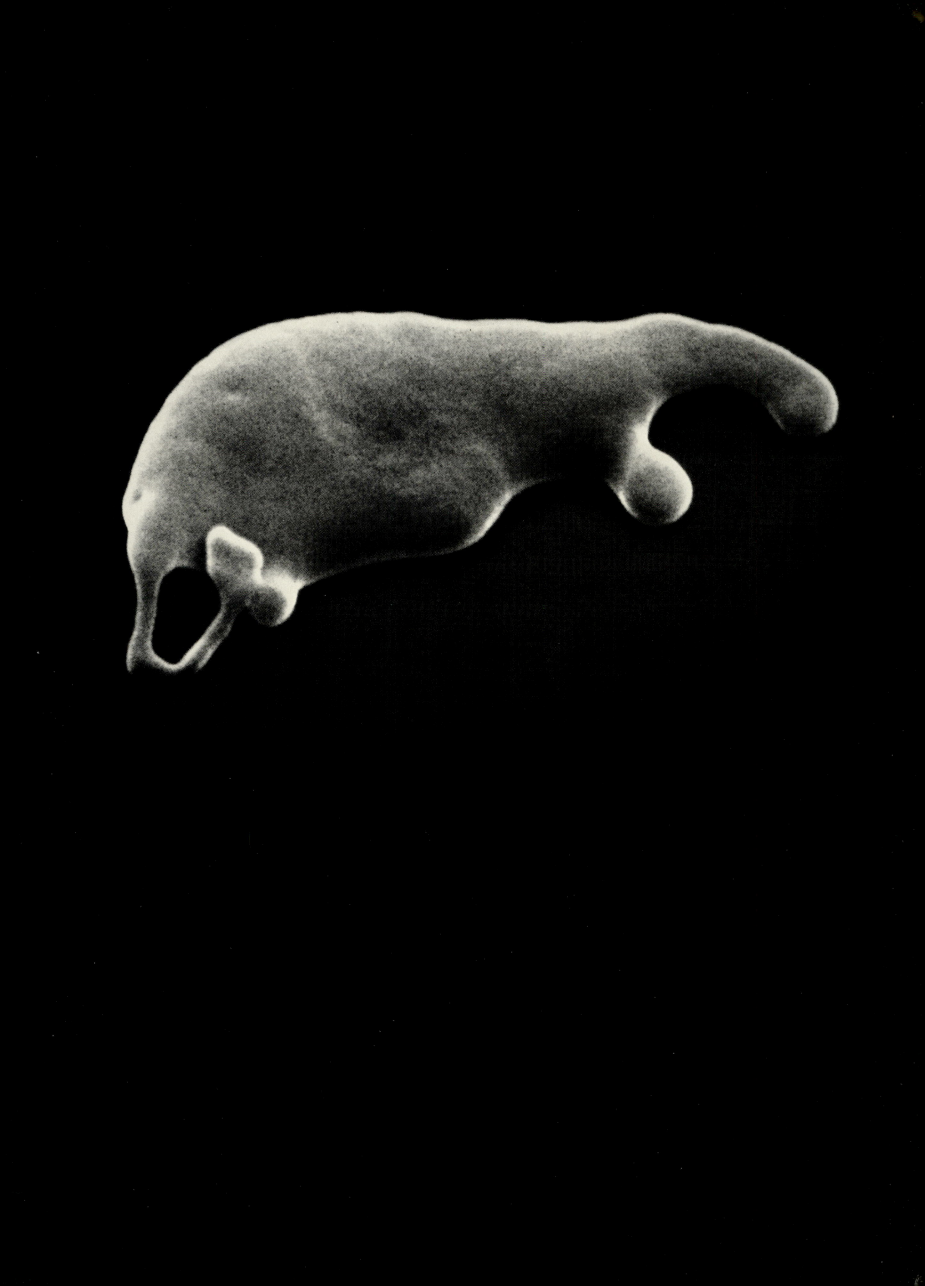

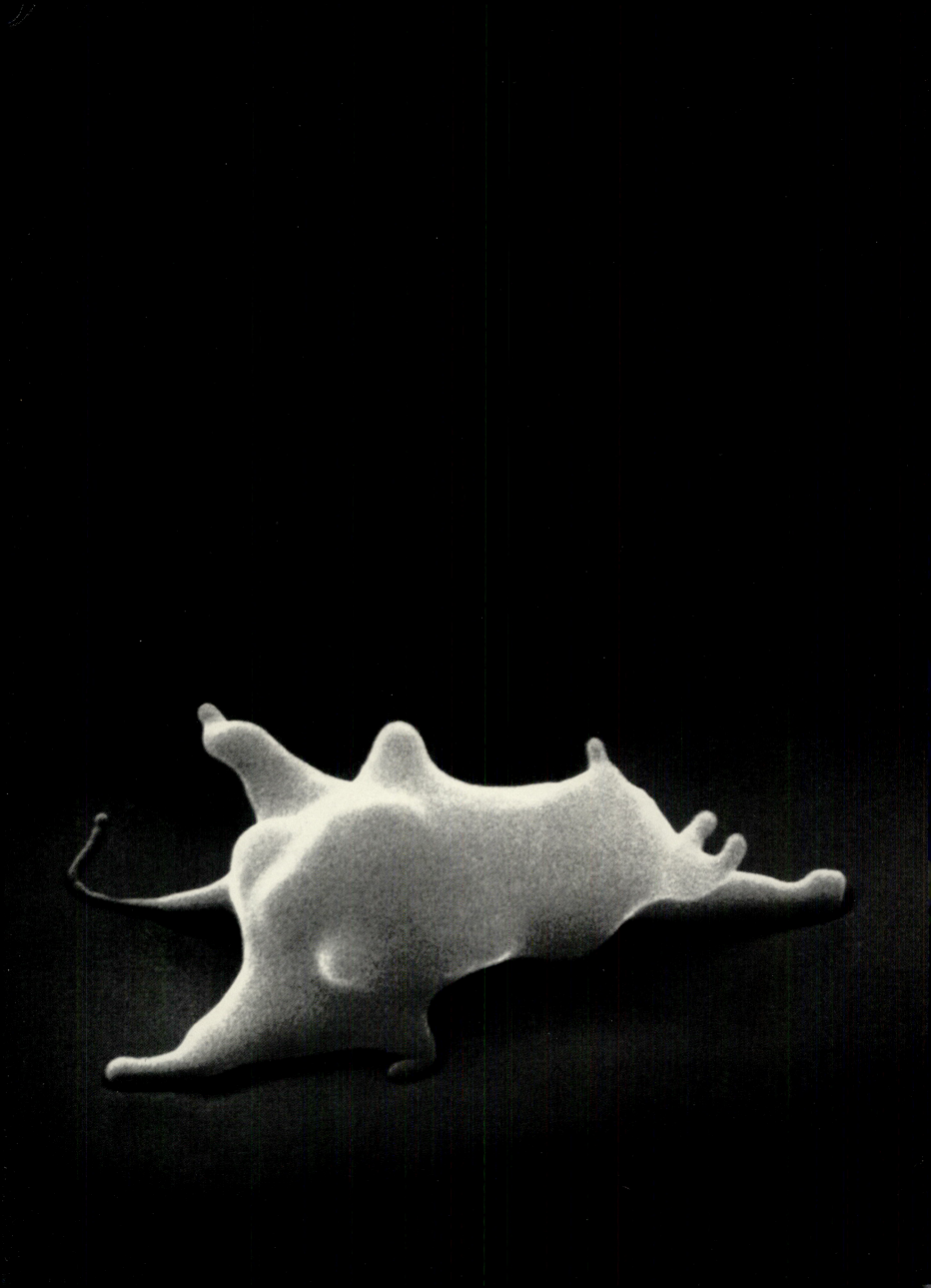

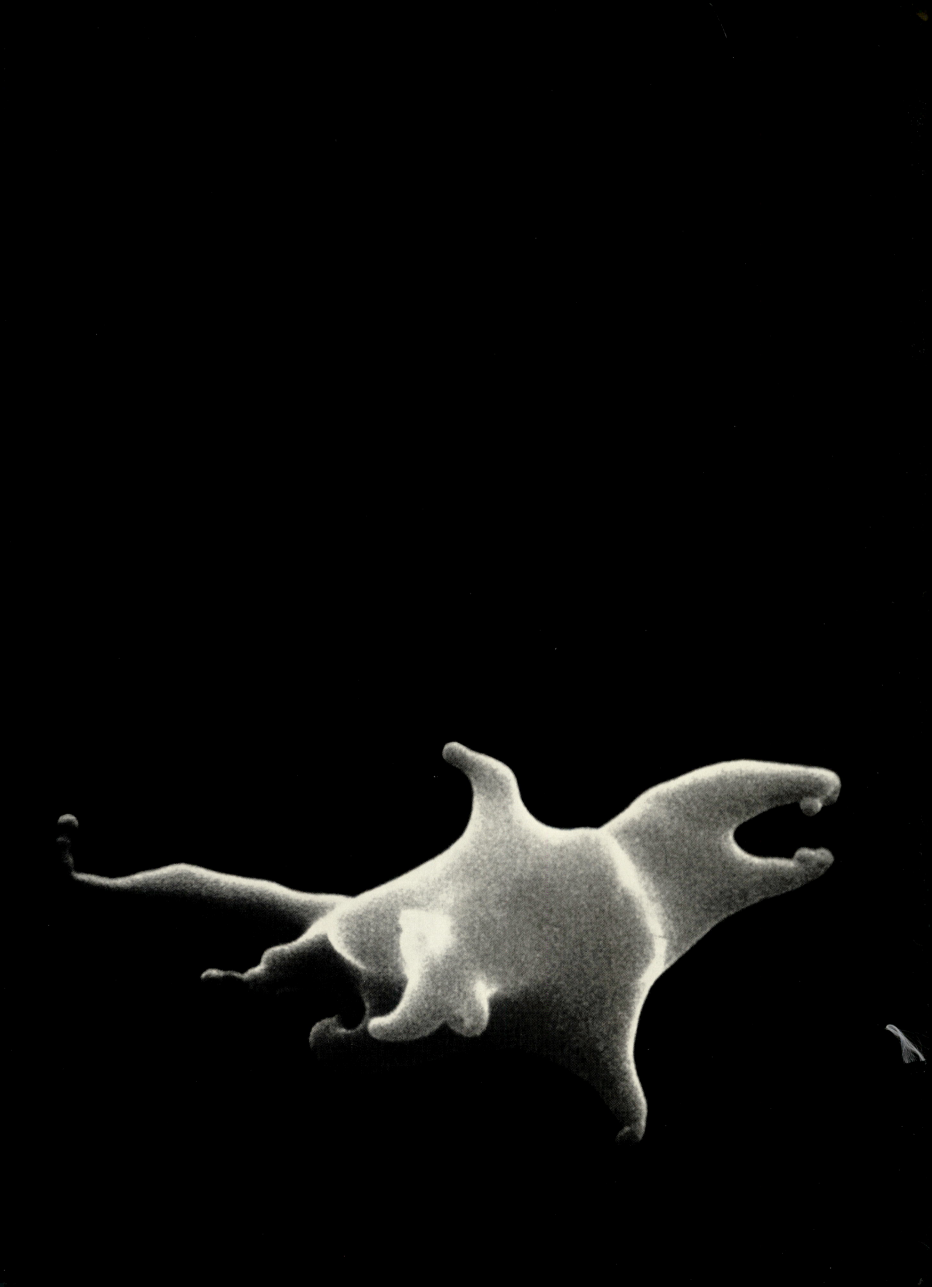

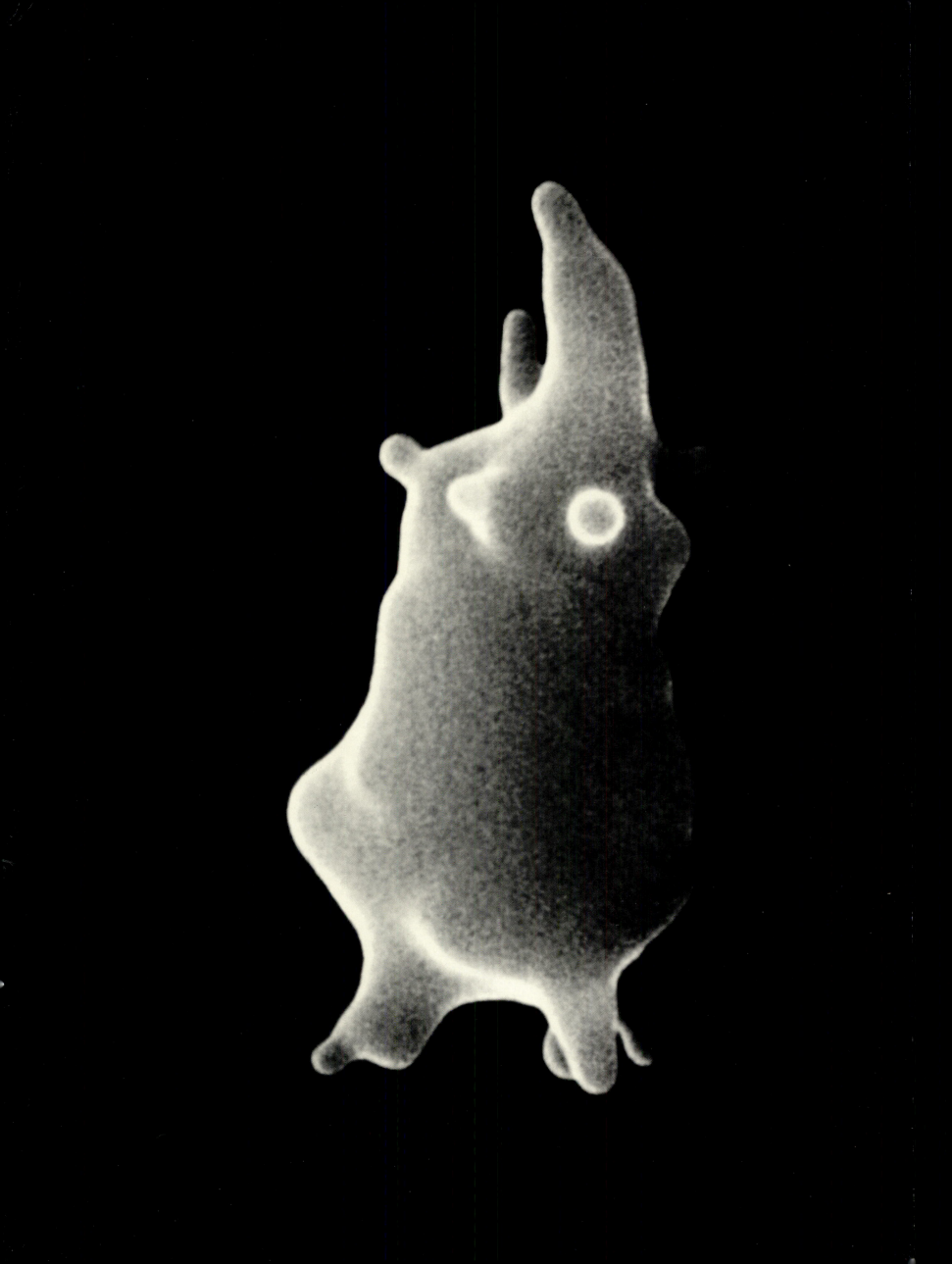

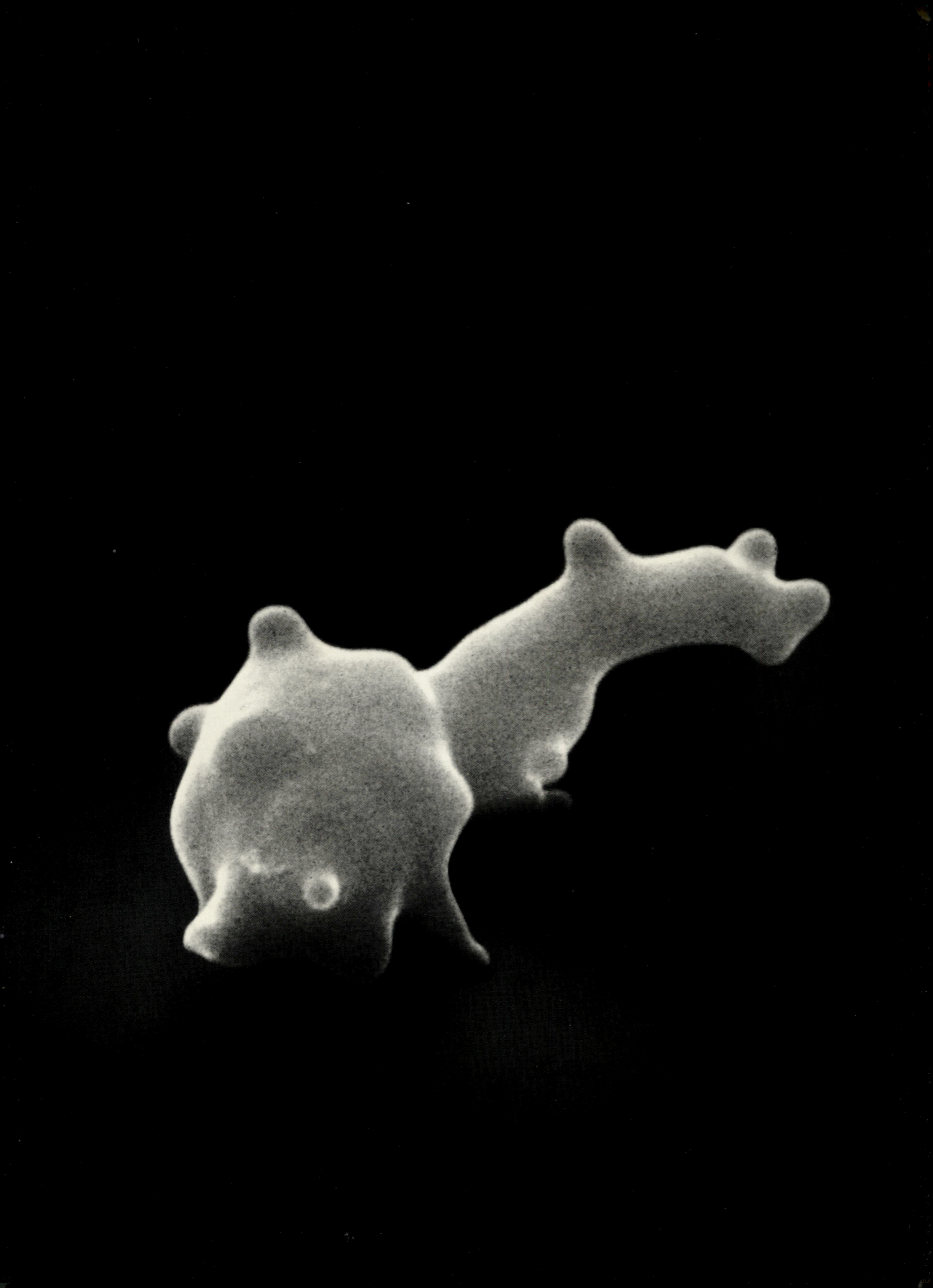

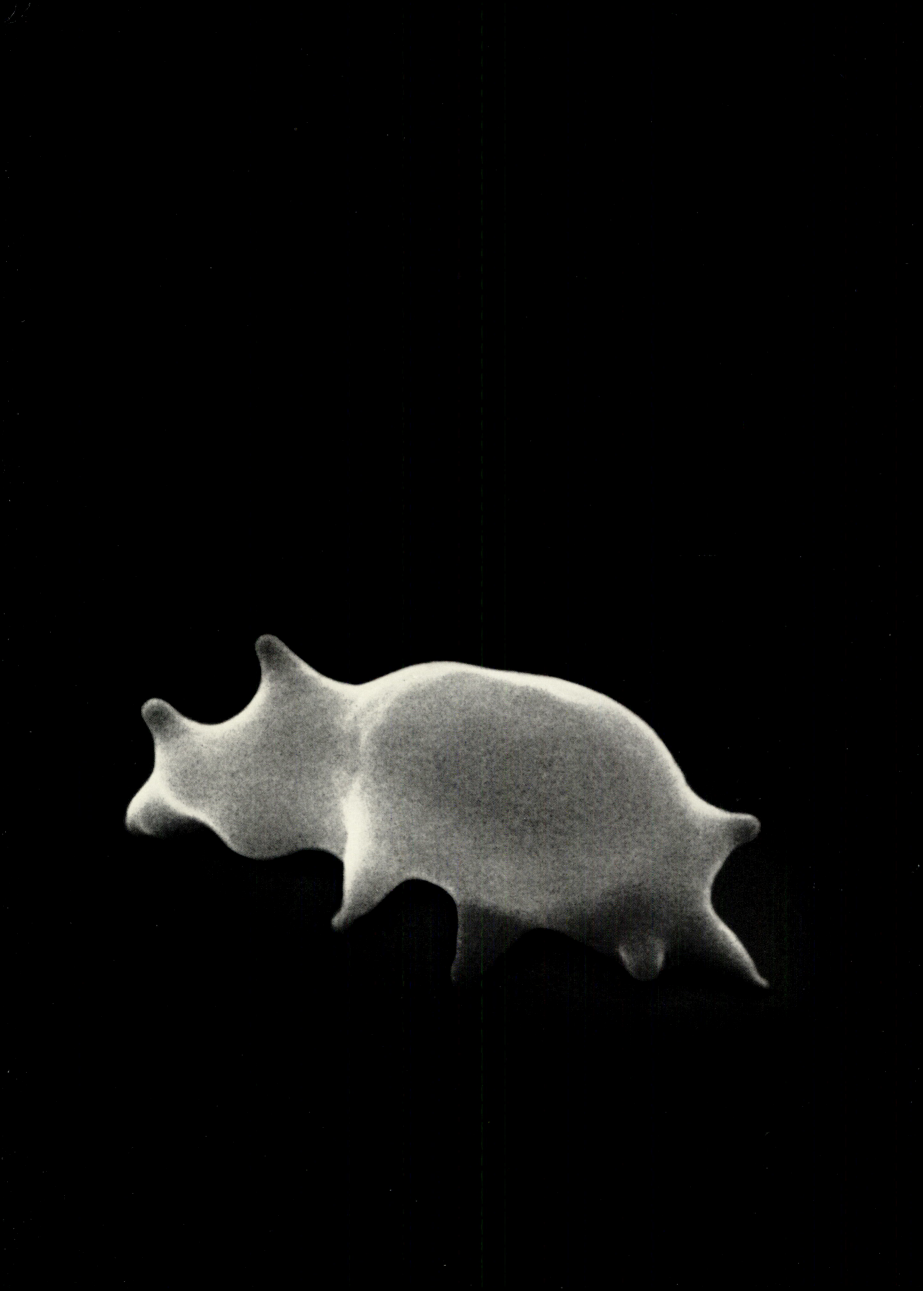

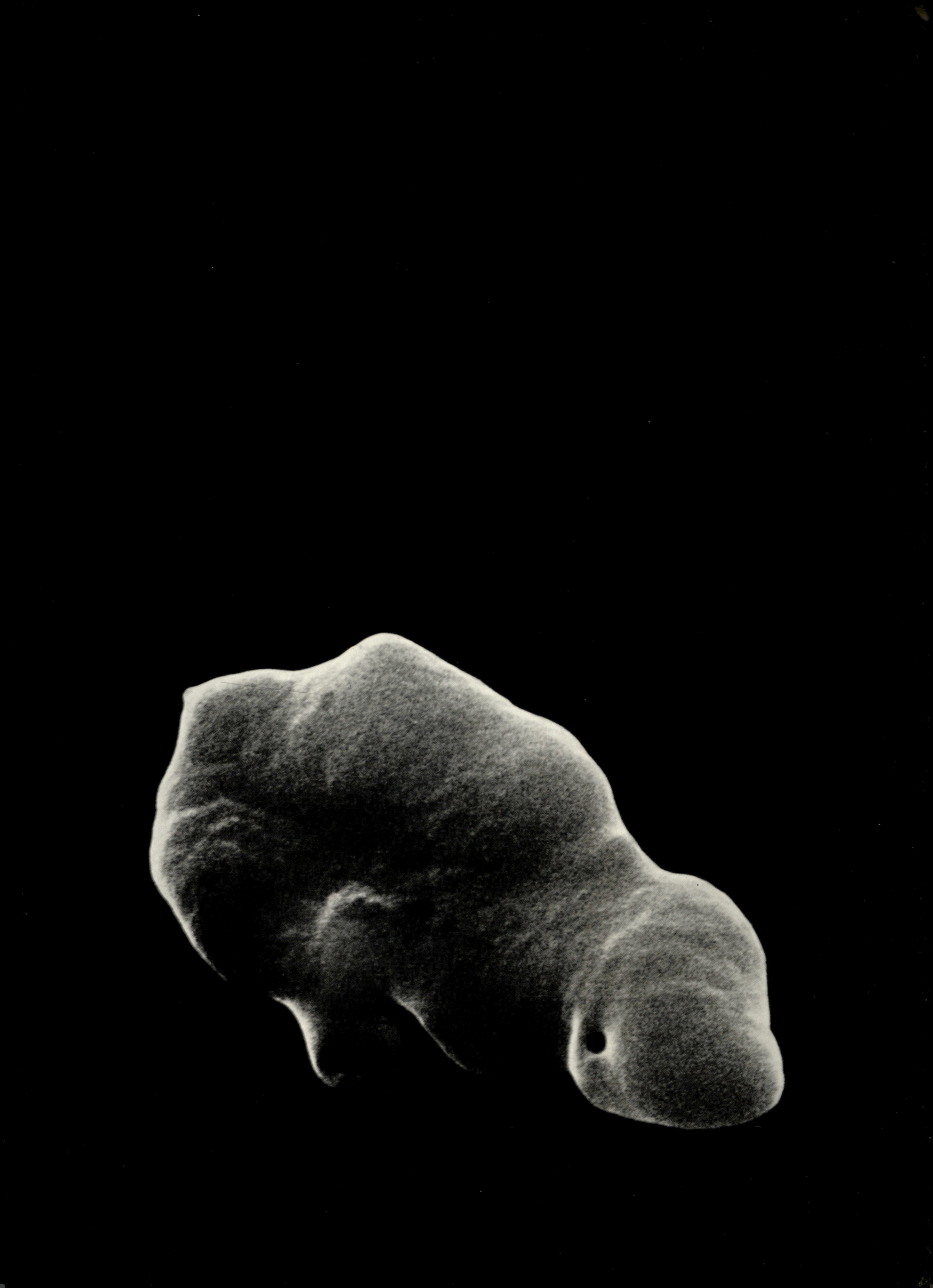

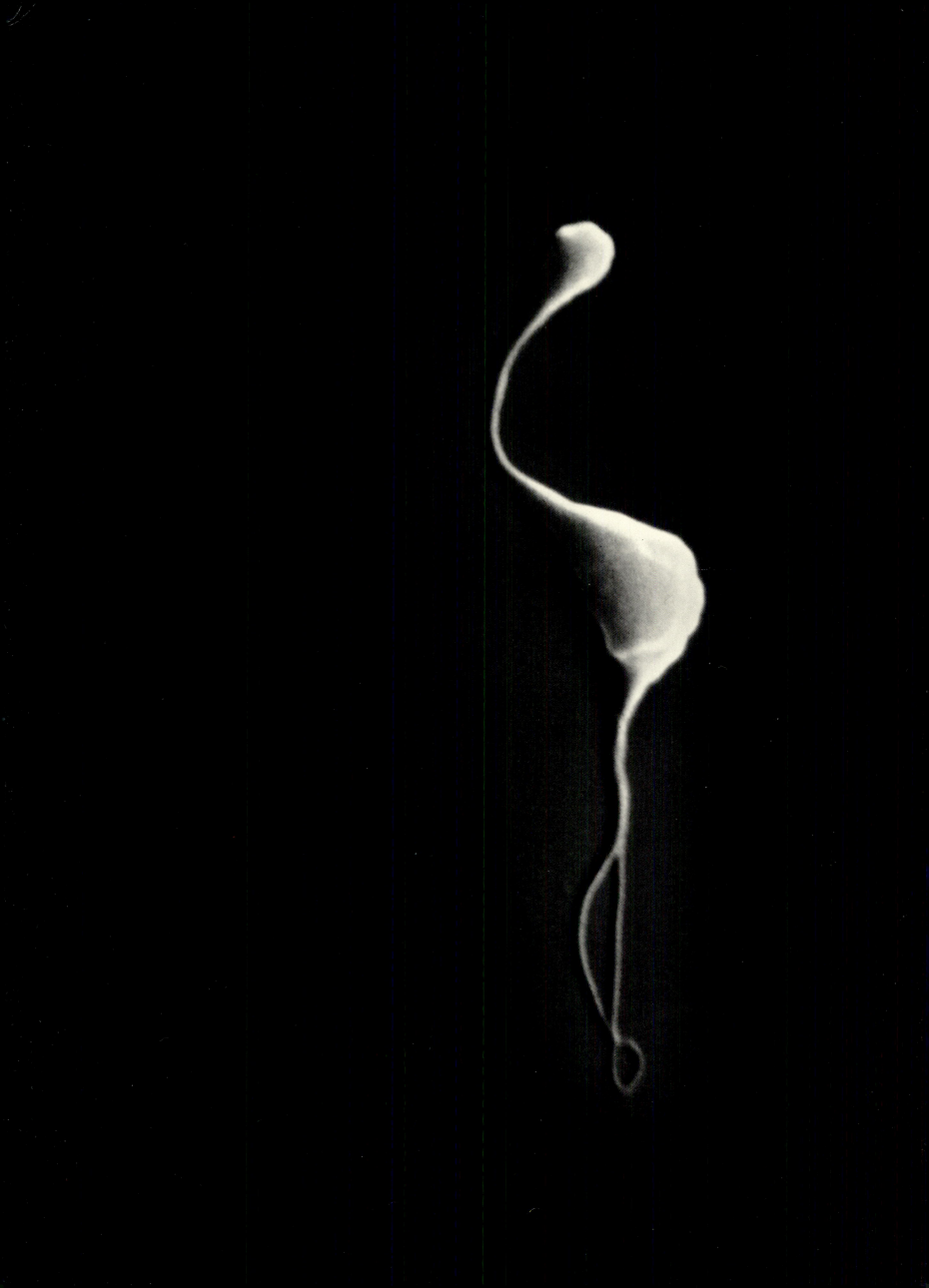

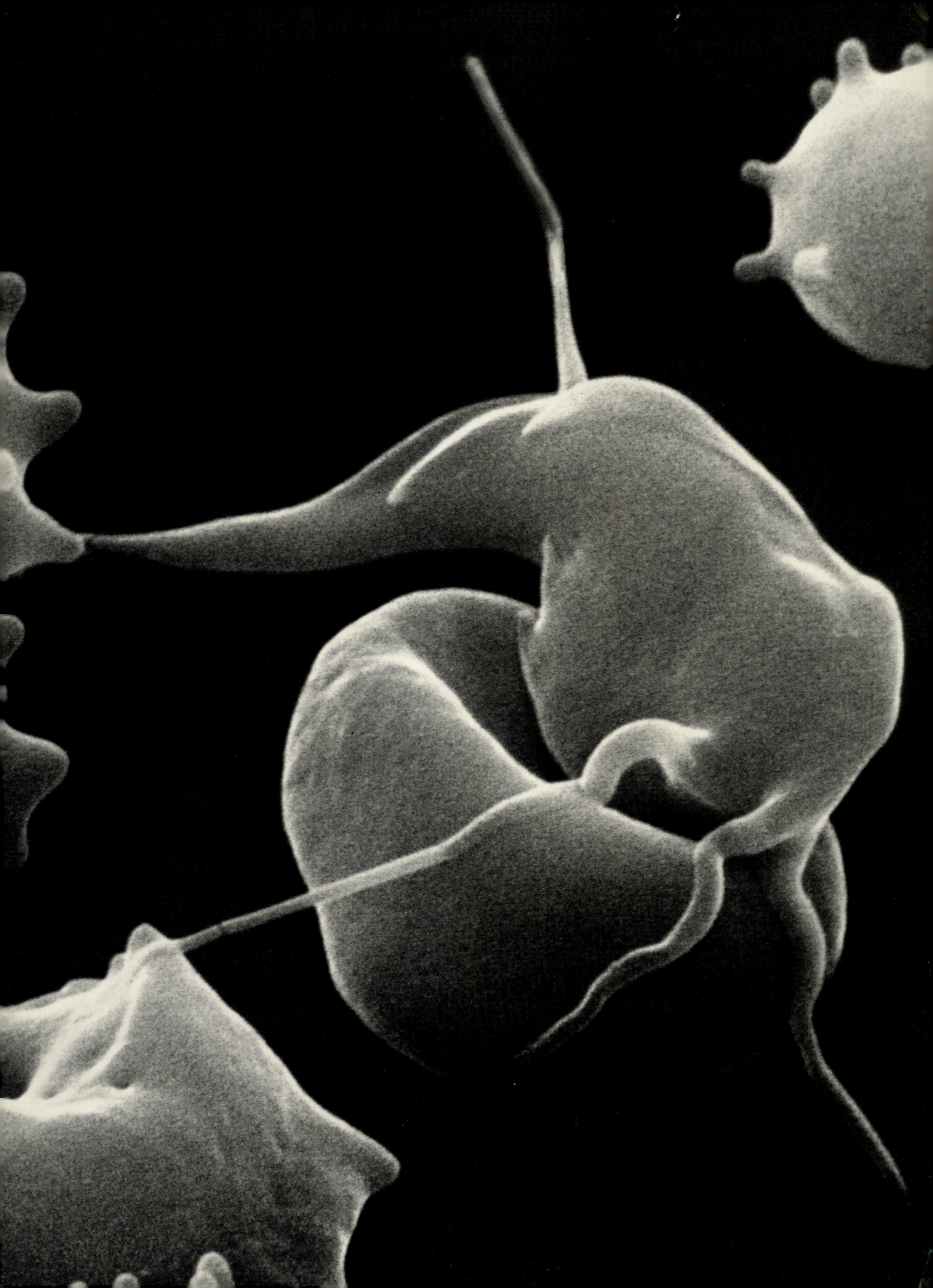

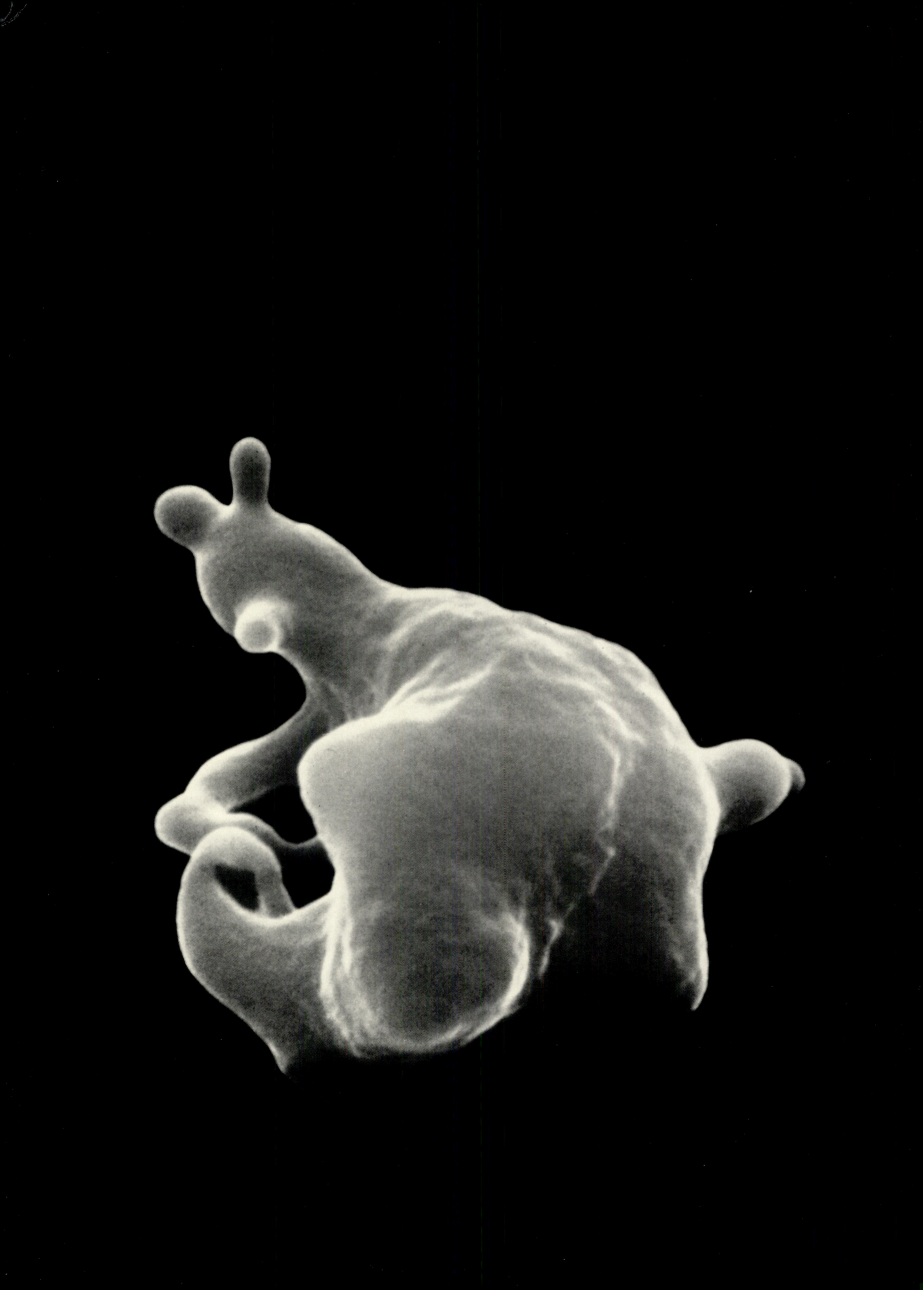

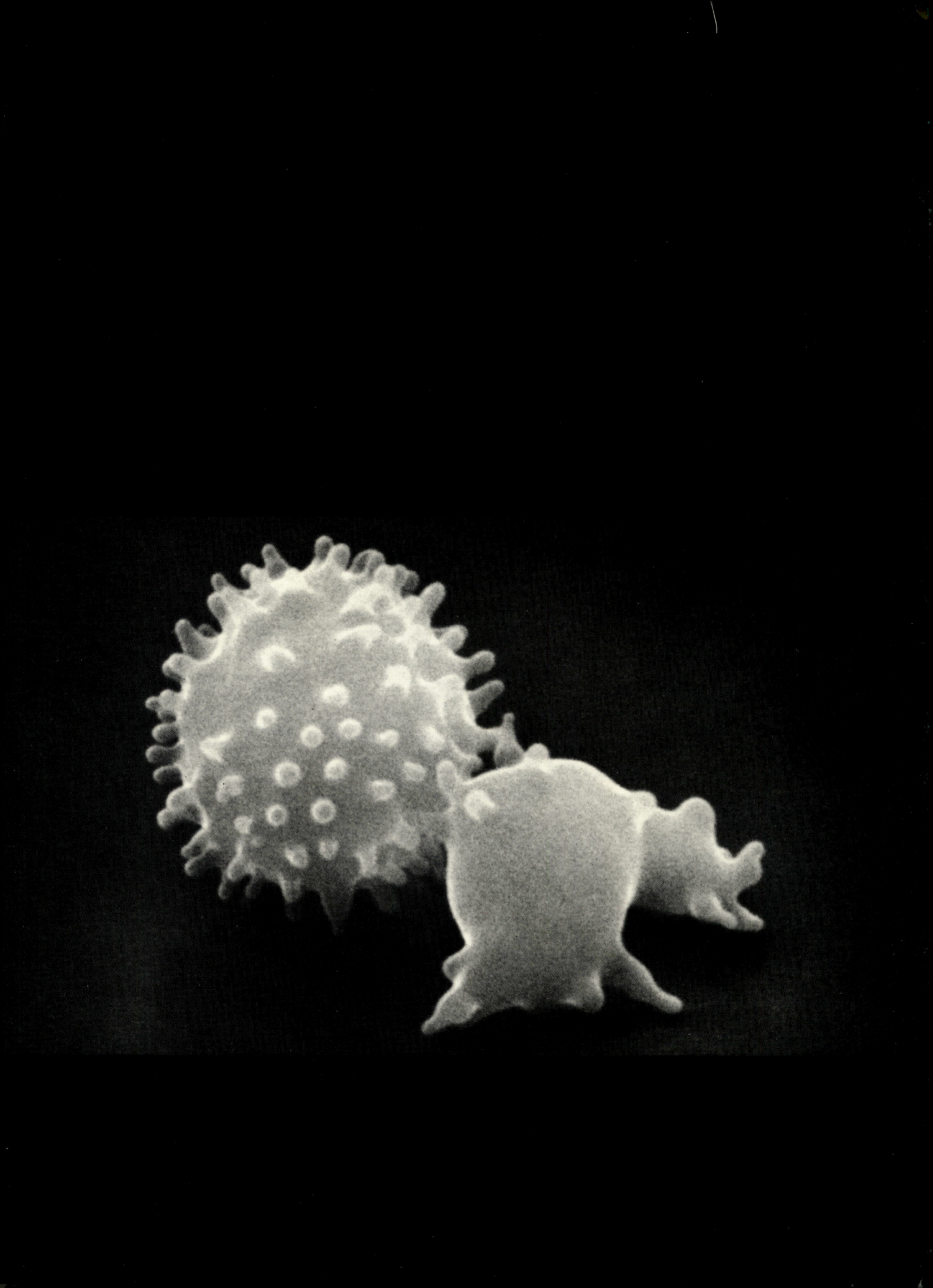

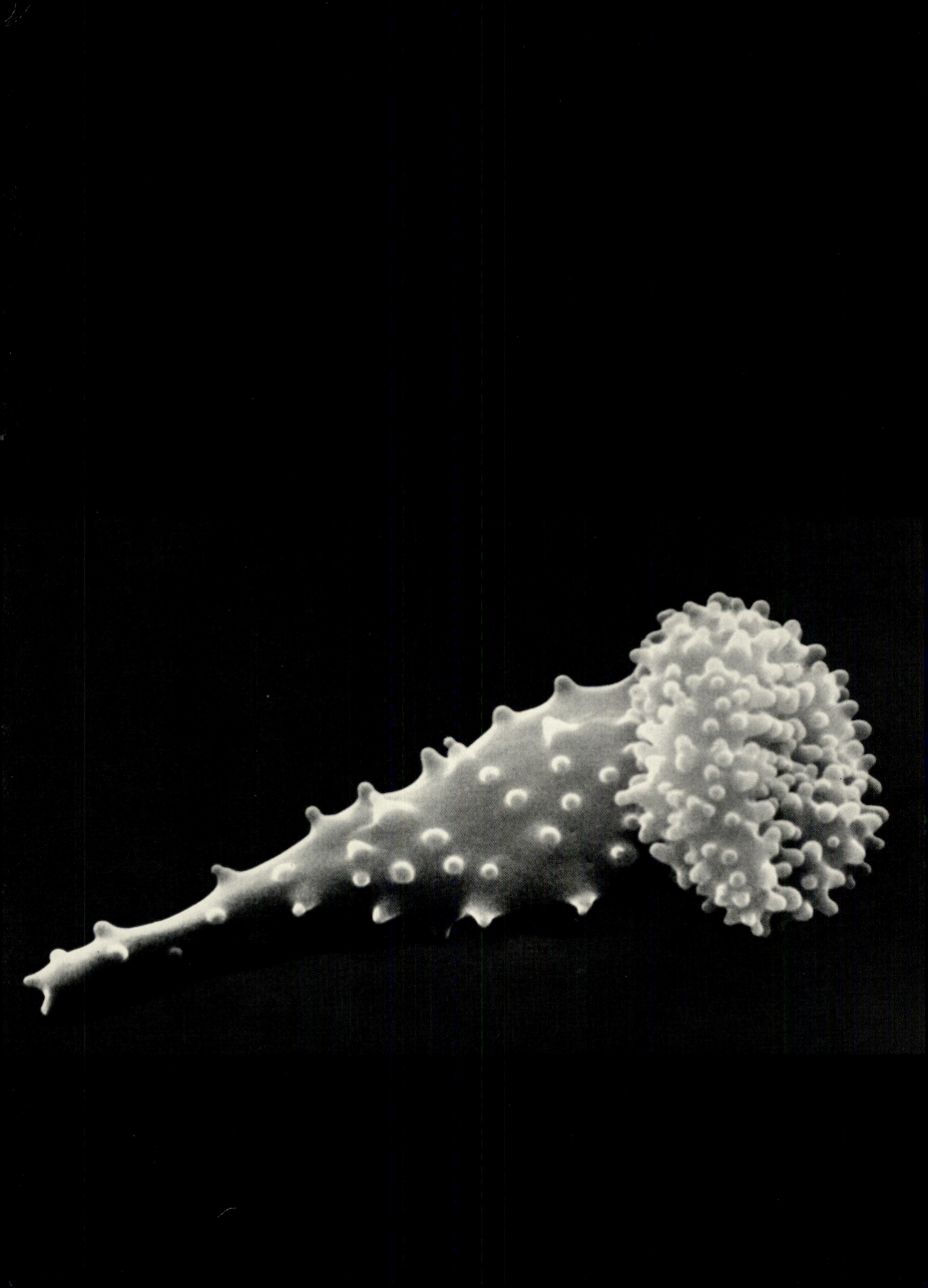

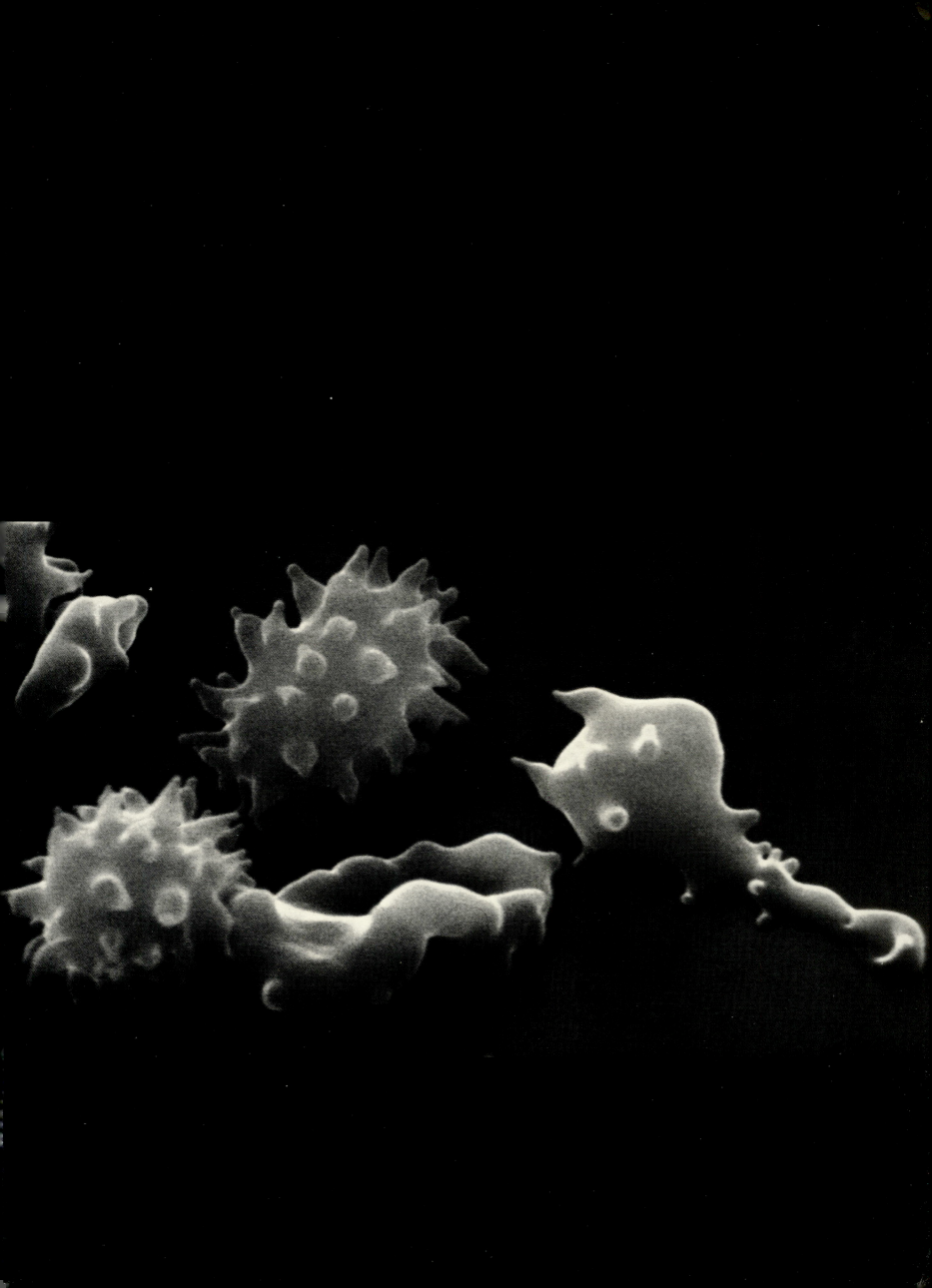

Chapter XIV

Micro-spherulation

Micro-spherulation

Red cells can lose fragments of different sizes, some large enough to be seen quite easily with the light microscope, others somewhat smaller and visible only with the electron microscope, still others so small as to be detectable only biochemically. This fragmentation occurs in response to changes in the micro-environment or intrinsic changes in the cell itself or both. It results in a decrease in the surface-to-volume ratio of the cell. If the process continues, the cell ultimately becomes spherical, hence no longer deformable, and lyses when passing through small capillaries.

The high lipid content of the red cell envelope is expressed morphologically by the appearance of microspherules and myelin figures in damaged cells. Myelin figures are curious morphological entities having the appearance of sinuous rods or filaments with bead-like swellings. Their name comes from their first being observed, in 1884, when myelin and water were mixed. Physicists have shown them to be equilibrium forms of anisotropic liquids such as lecithin of phosphatides mixed with water.

Red cells stored for a long period of time will first undergo the echinocytic transformation and then fragment by budding and produce microspherules and myelin figures. These may remain attached to the erythrocyte and particularly the spicules on the echinocyte surface. More often they detach themselves, and when observed in a drop of blood, they appear to be animated by a Brownian movement; at times they have been mistaken for micro-organisms.

Fig. 1. Echinocytes in aged blood. Beginning microspherulation of spicules.

Figs. 2 and 3. Myelin figures arising from spicules of sphero-echinocytes. They can be tubular or "strings of pearls" and can become detached and float free in the plasma.

Fig. 4. Isolated myelin figures, from aged blood, separated by ultracentrifugation. Their shape has been preserved by the freeze-drying method.

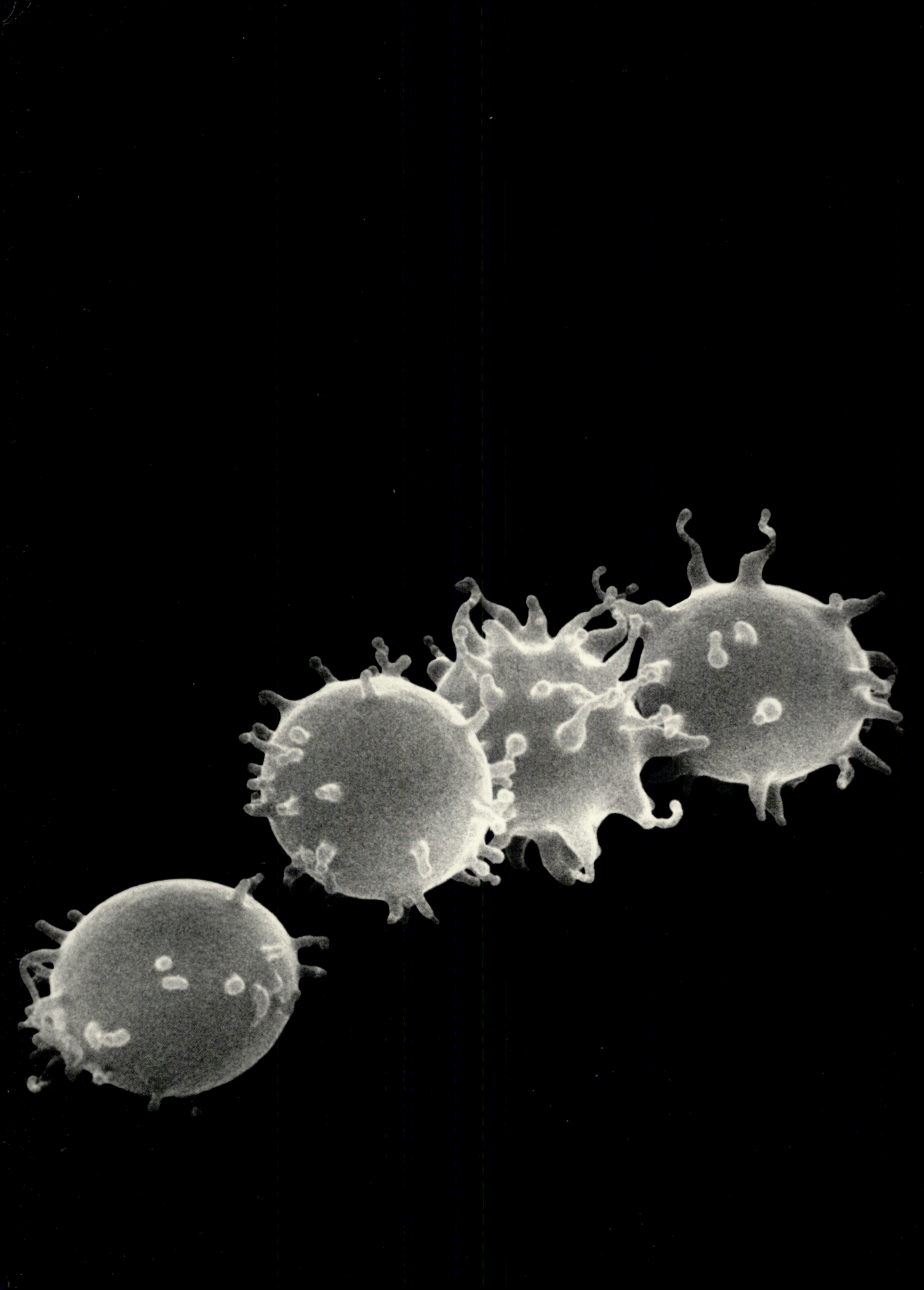

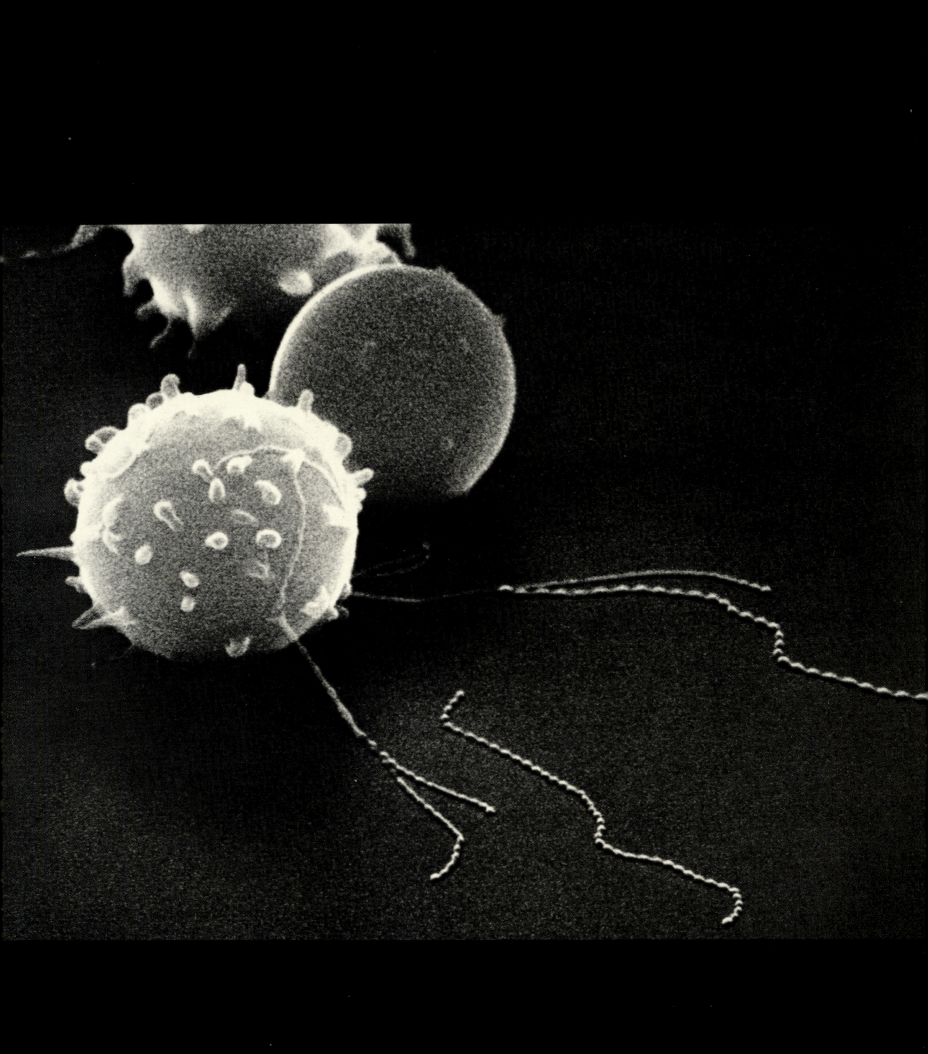

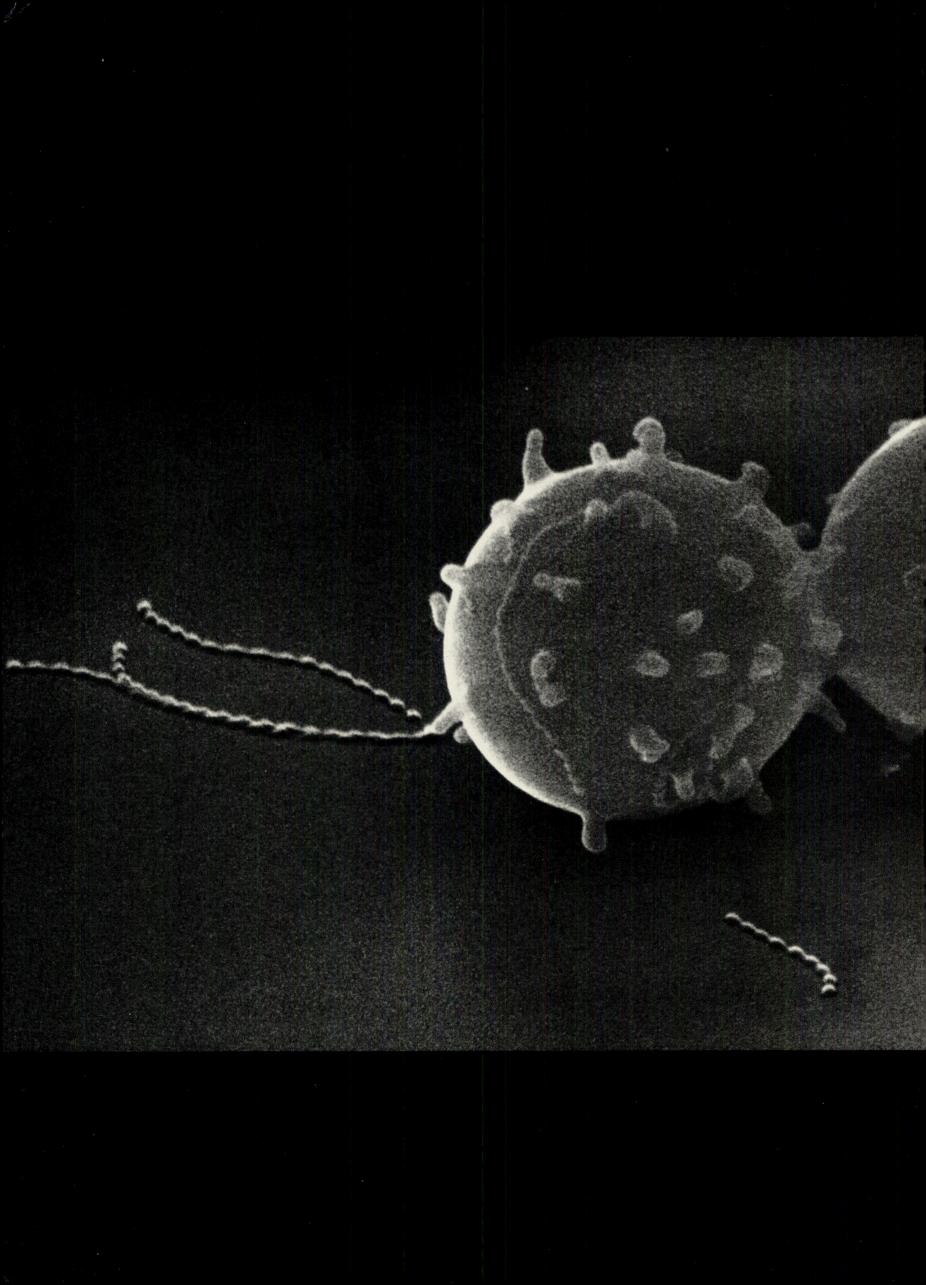

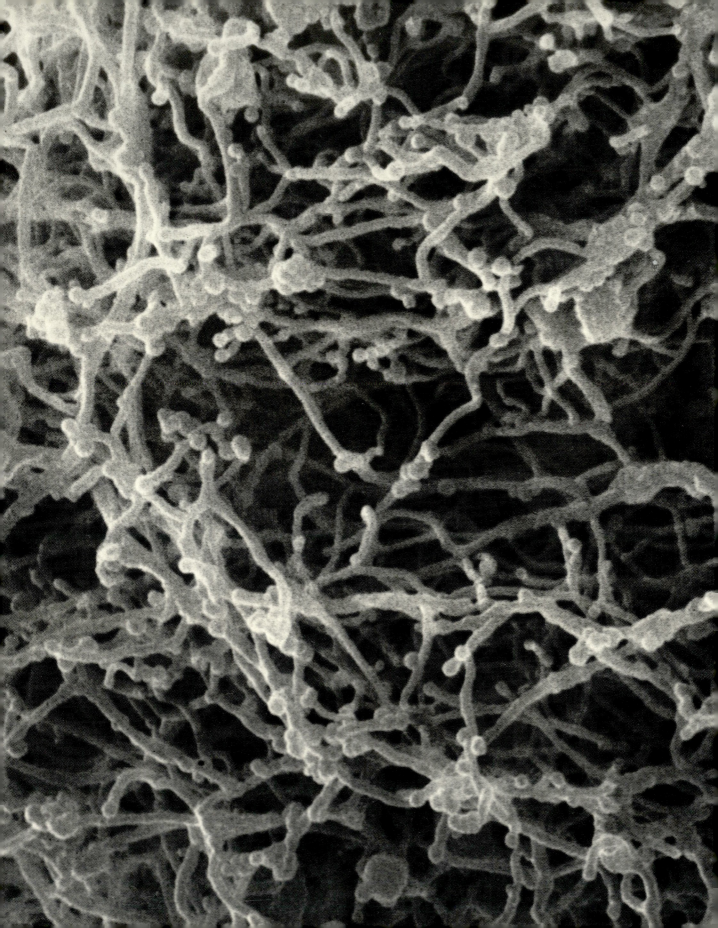

Chapter XV

Hemolysis

Hemolysis

Hemolysis is the loss of hemoglobin from red cells. It leaves the "ghost" of a cell behind. It is a result of physical or chemical injuries or of the action of antibodies or of a hypotonic medium. In these circumstances, the red cell takes up water and swells to the limit dictated by the elasticity of its membrane. When the cell reaches a critical volume (175% of normal for discocytes, though the figure may vary greatly in disease) the hemoglobin escapes and hemolysis occurs.

Hemolysis by antibodies requires the presence of Complement. As few as 30 molecules of certain antibodies may cause the lysis of a red blood cell, but 6,000 molecules of complement are needed. Chemical substances which may lyse red cells include saponin, fatty acids, bile salts, lysolecithin, and many poisons: snake venoms, benzol, and bacterial toxins.

If the red blood cells are subjected to pressure, e.g., pressure of the coverslip on a thinly spread fresh drop of blood, hemolysis ensues. In this connection a surprising form of hemolytic anemia may be cited. The hemoglobinuria in certain athletes after a foot-race or a game of jai alai is the result of damage to red blood cells within the capillaries at the site of the pressure.

Echinocytes and discocytes, having passed through a spherical form prior to hemolysis, resume their echinocytic or discocytic shape after lysis.

Fig. 1. Pre-hemolytic sphero-echinocyte.

Fig. 2. Sphero-echinocytes in various stages of pre-hemolysis.

Fig. 3. Sphero-echinocytes. Steps between sphero-echinocytes and spherocytes.

Figs. 4, 5, and 6. Ghosts, after hemolysis.

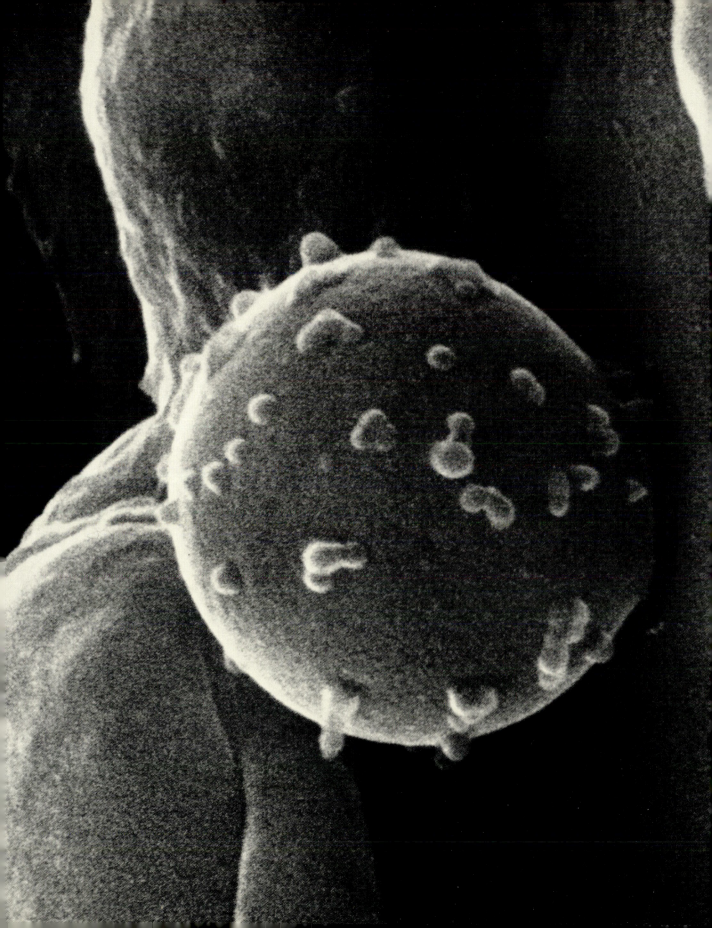

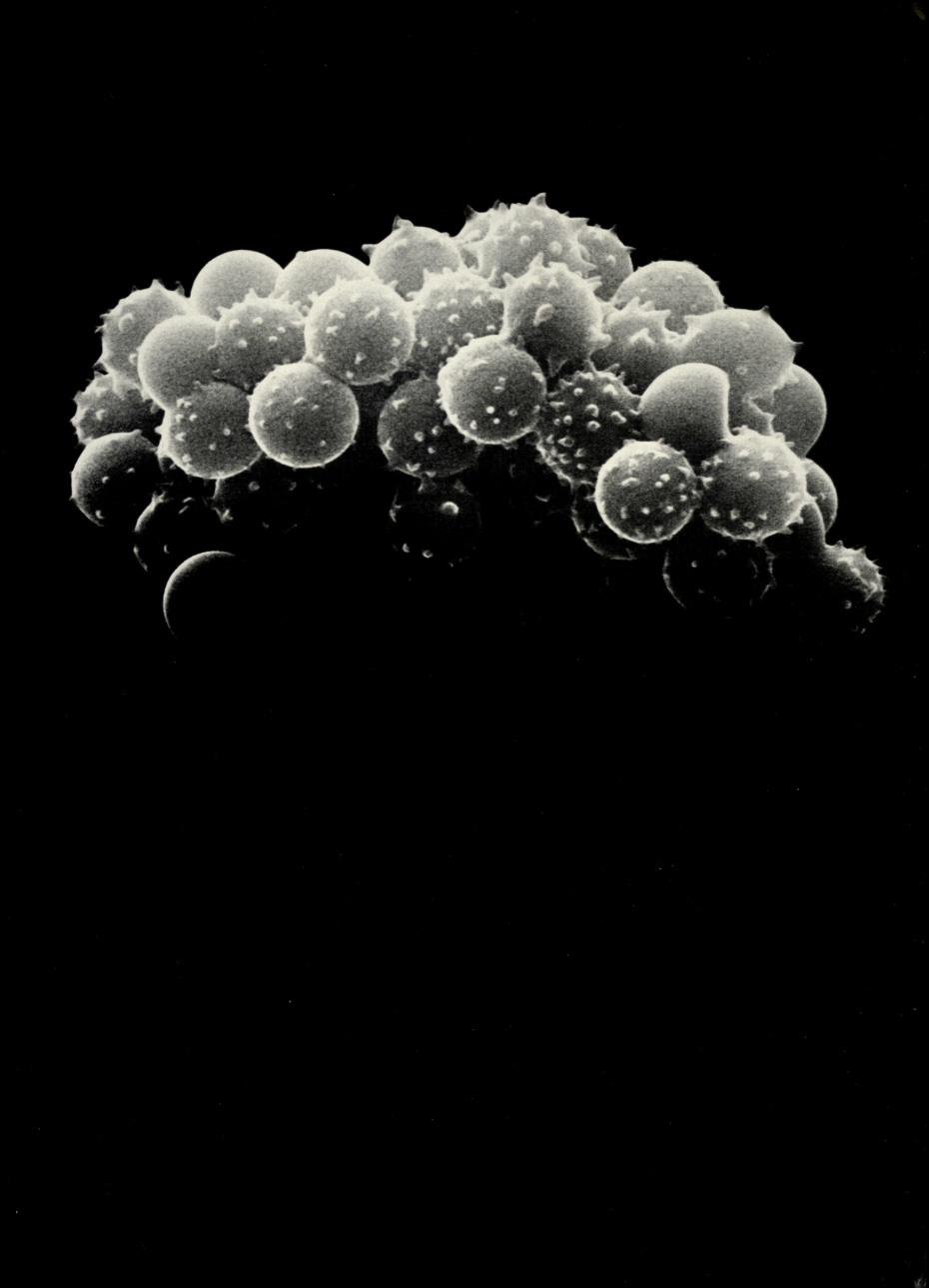

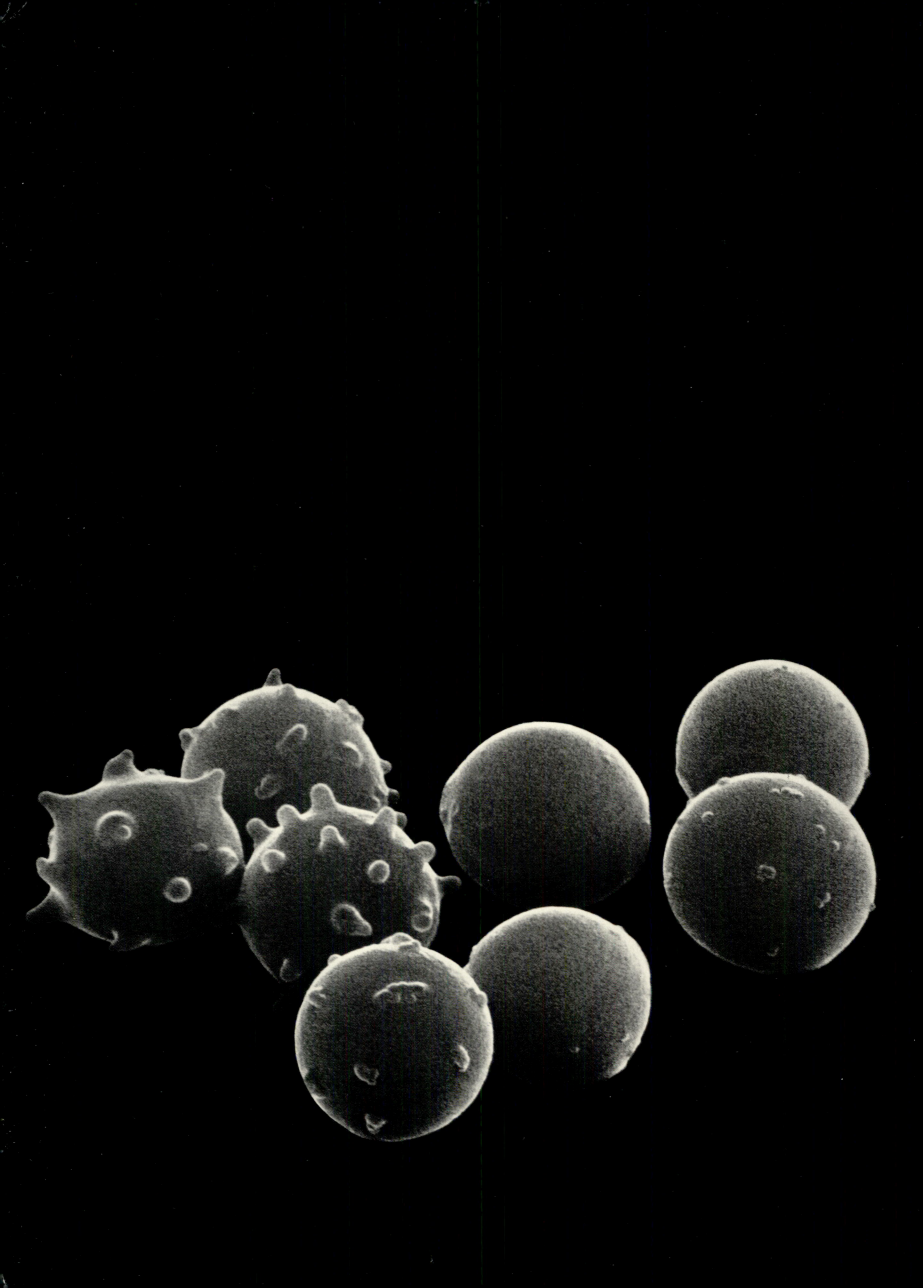

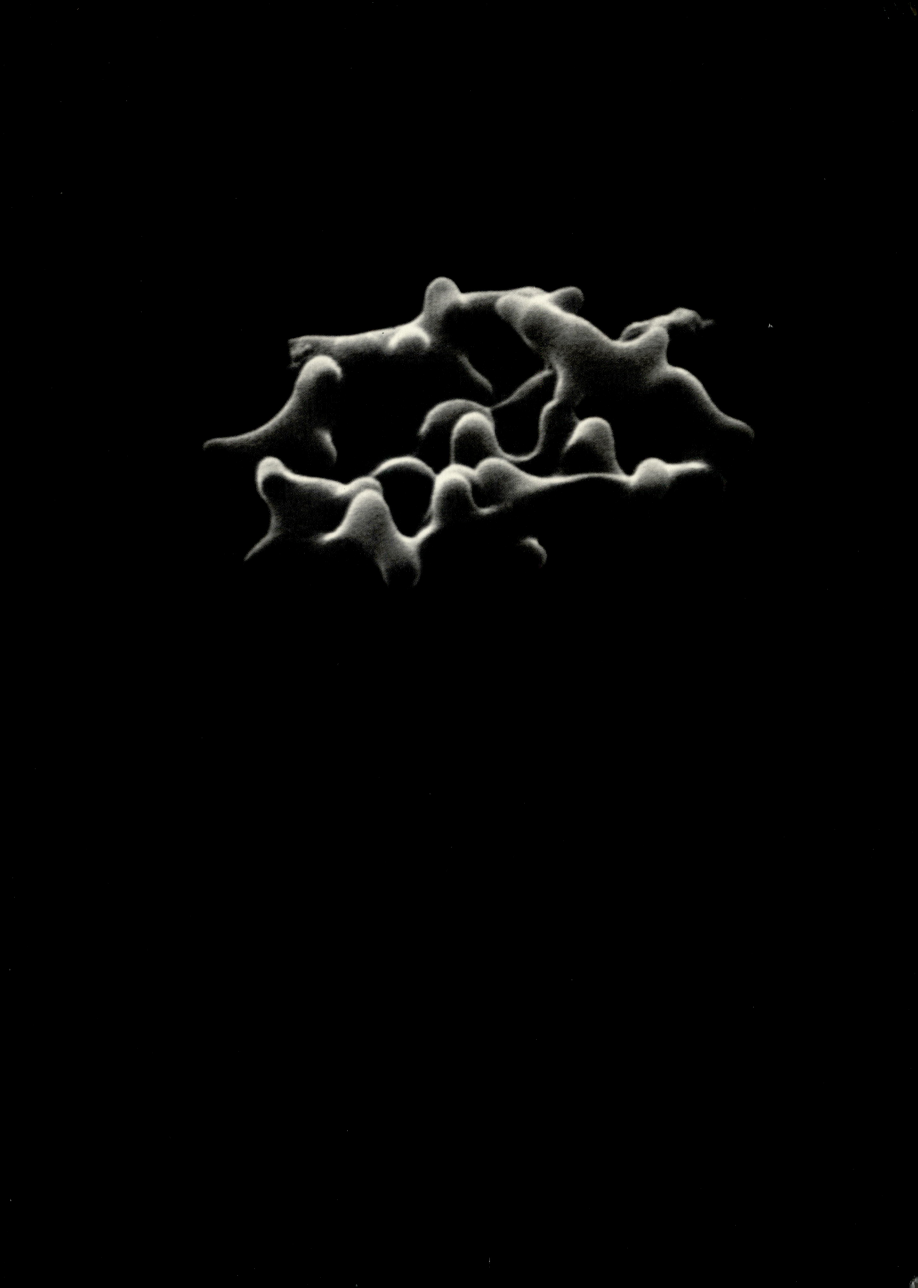

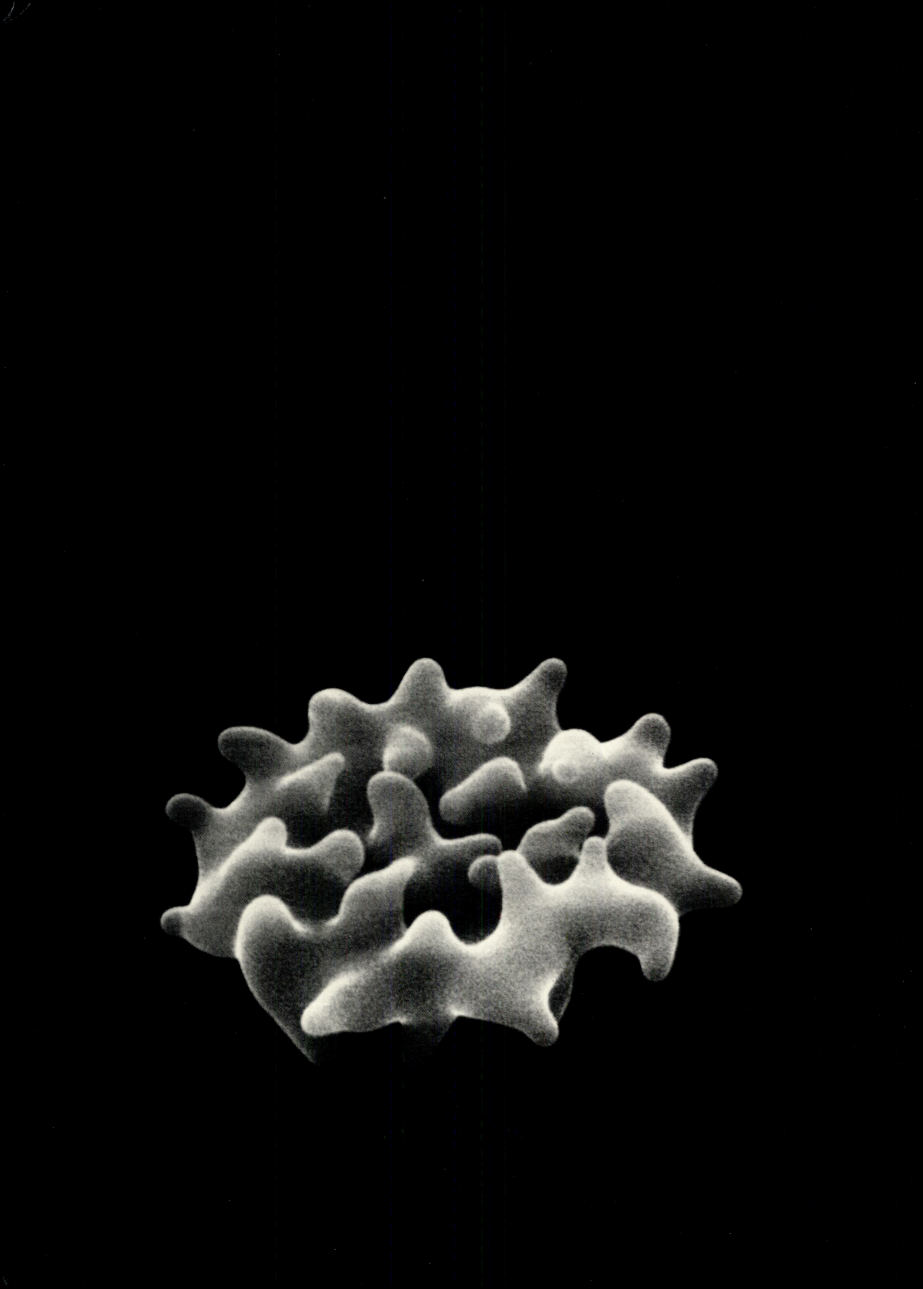

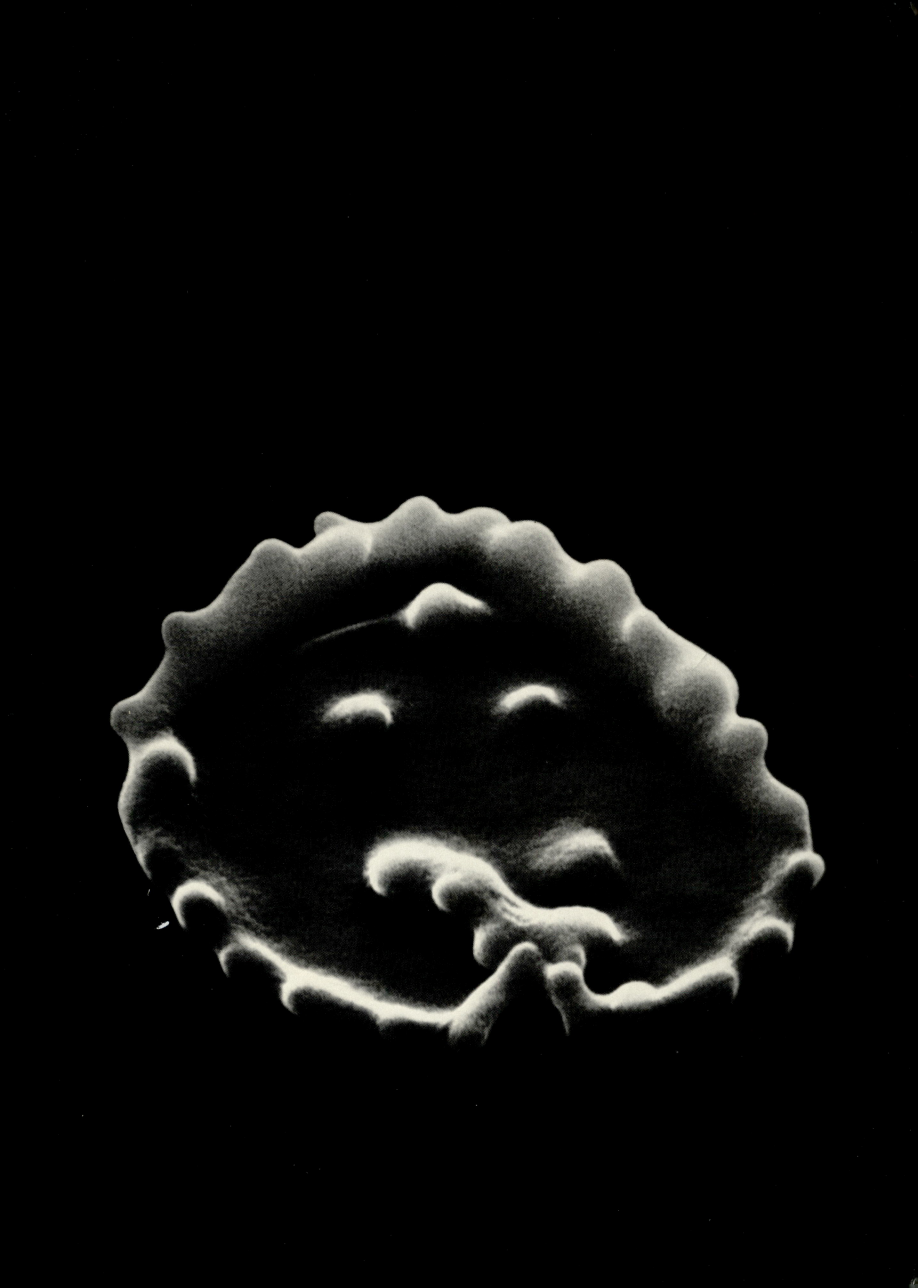

Chapter XVI

Red Cell Death

Red Cell Death

Like all living creatures, the red blood cell comes to its natural end in death. The moment of death, like conception, birth, maturation, and function of the cell, is planned and governed by an inexorable mechanism. In a normal human being, only red cells which have reached an age of about 110 days disappear from the bloodstream. The aging process may be due to internal depletions, the exhaustion of metabolic or enzyme reserves which cannot be replenished, or external wear and the gradual deterioration of the cell membrane caused by mechanical or chemical injuries. It may also be caused by the gradual accumulation of unavoidable errors in the molecular functions of the cell. At any rate, the cells which have reached old age disappear from the bloodstream.

A microscopist, a biophysicist, a biochemist cannot yet tell just what characterizes an old red cell, but a macrophage will recognize it immediately. It will throw out its veils in the direction of the aged cell, drag it off, envelop it, engulf it, and digest it.

Fig. 1. Attachment of macrophages to red cells and the first stage of phago-cytosis. On the left, poly-erythrophagocytosis. On the right, a macro-phage in the instant preceding phagocytosis, showing its funnel-shaped "mouth."

Figs. 2 and 3. Poly-erythrophagocytosis. This phenomenon is quite frequent; the phagocytic cells extend veils in several directions and can phago-cytosize several cells at the same time. Note that all the discocytes have become spherocytes.

Fig. 4. Fastening on to the prey.

Figs. 5, 6, and 7. Stages of the engulfment.

Fig. 8. Engulfment completed and beginning of digestion.

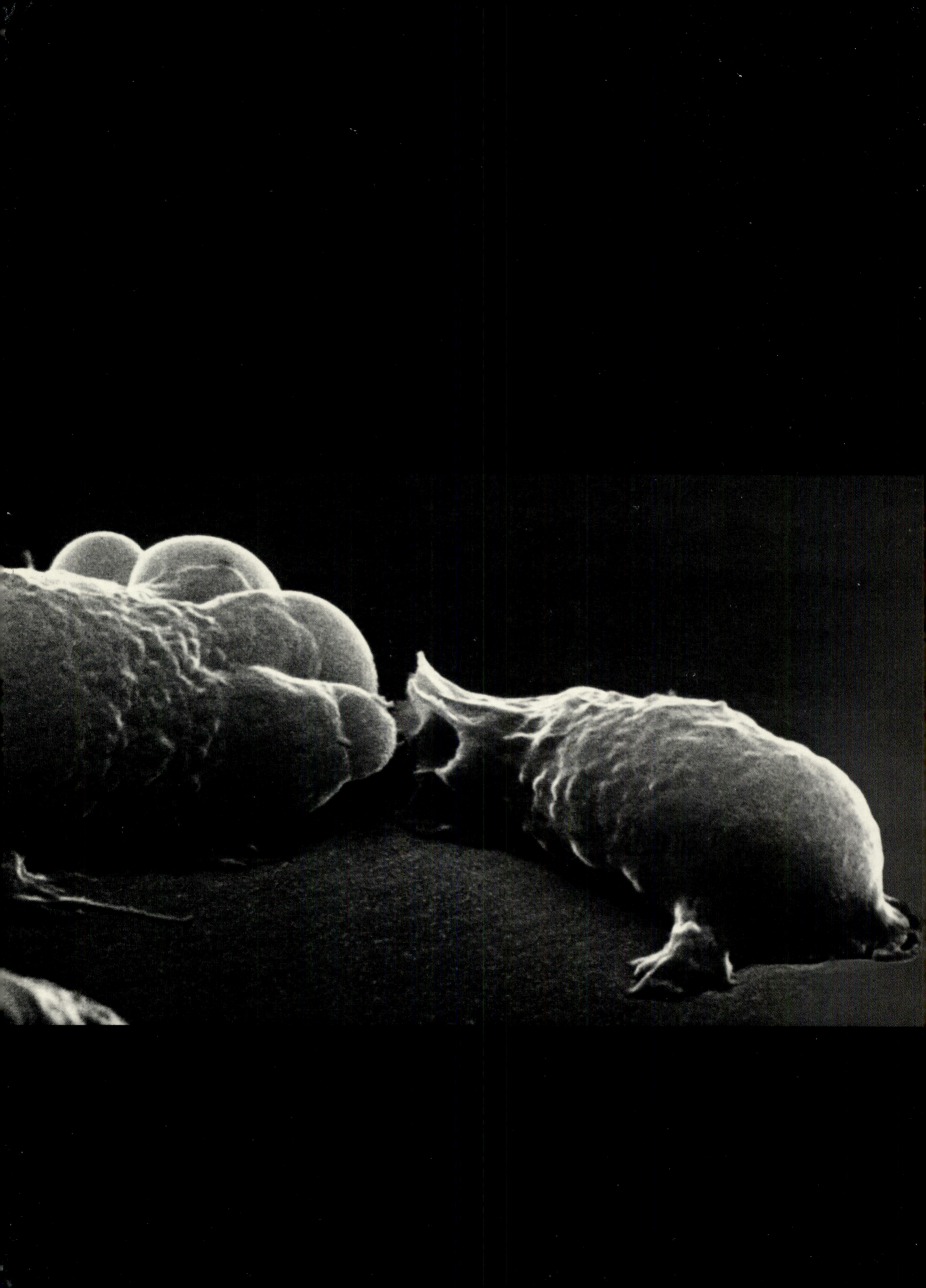

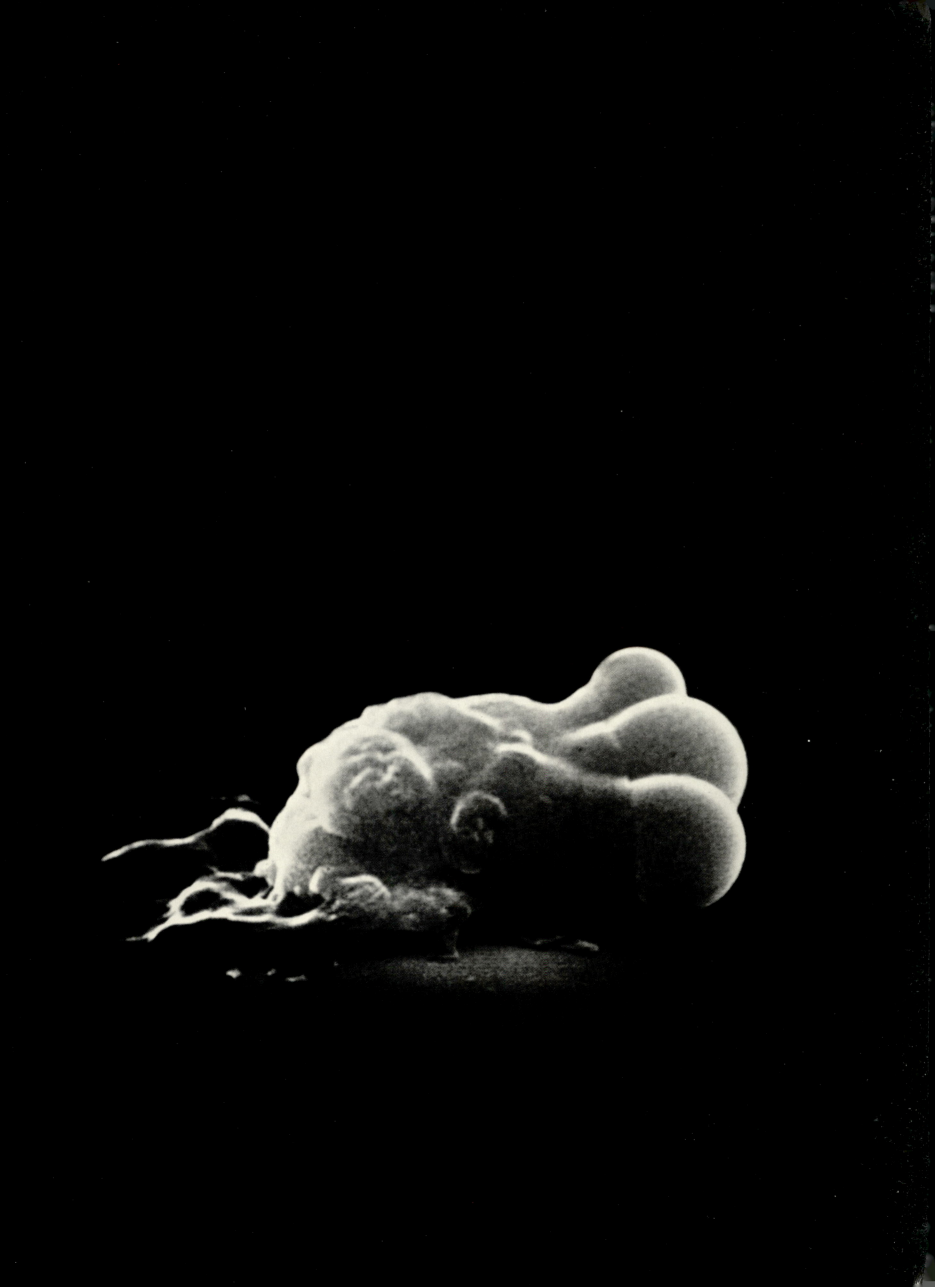

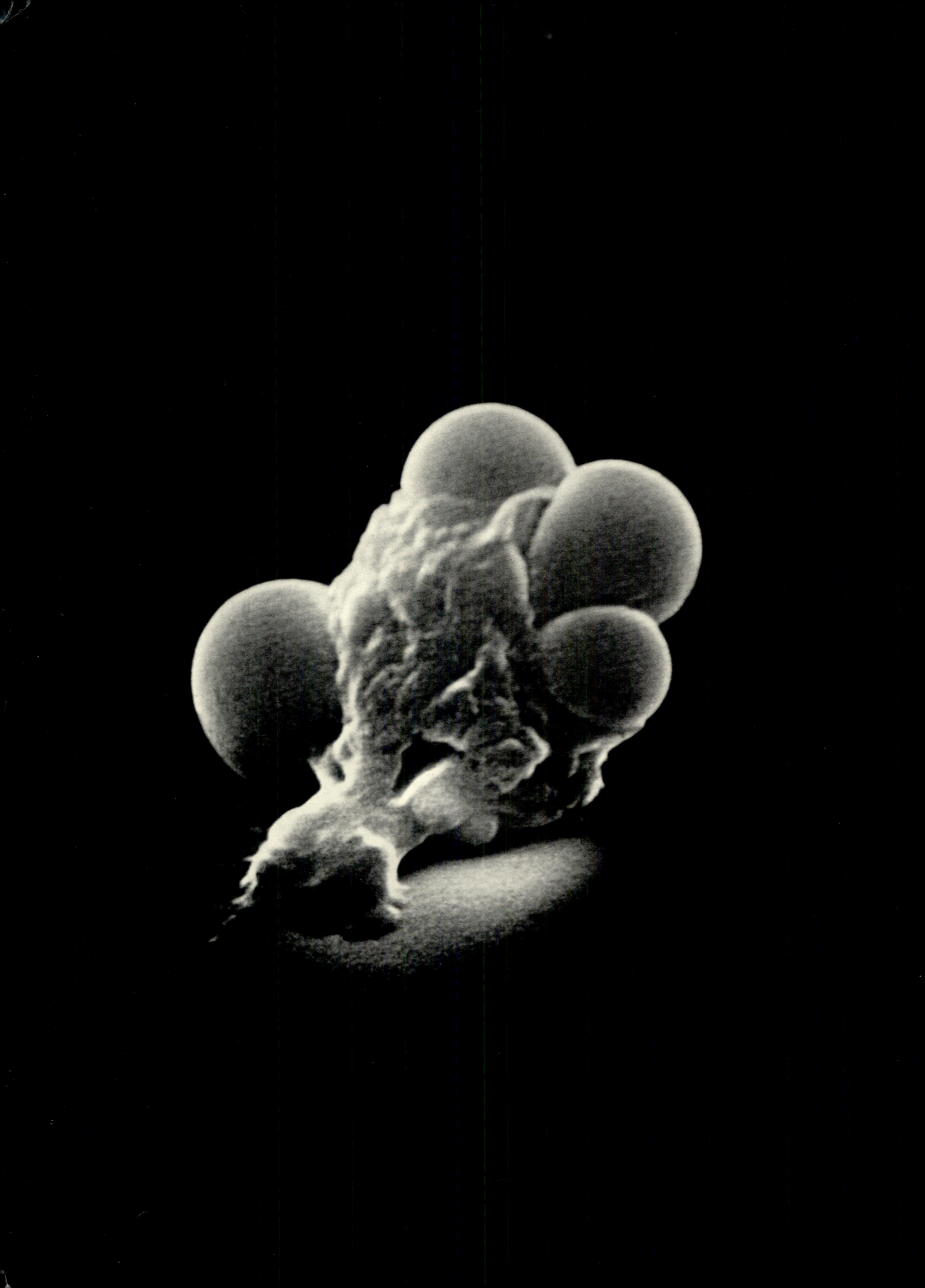

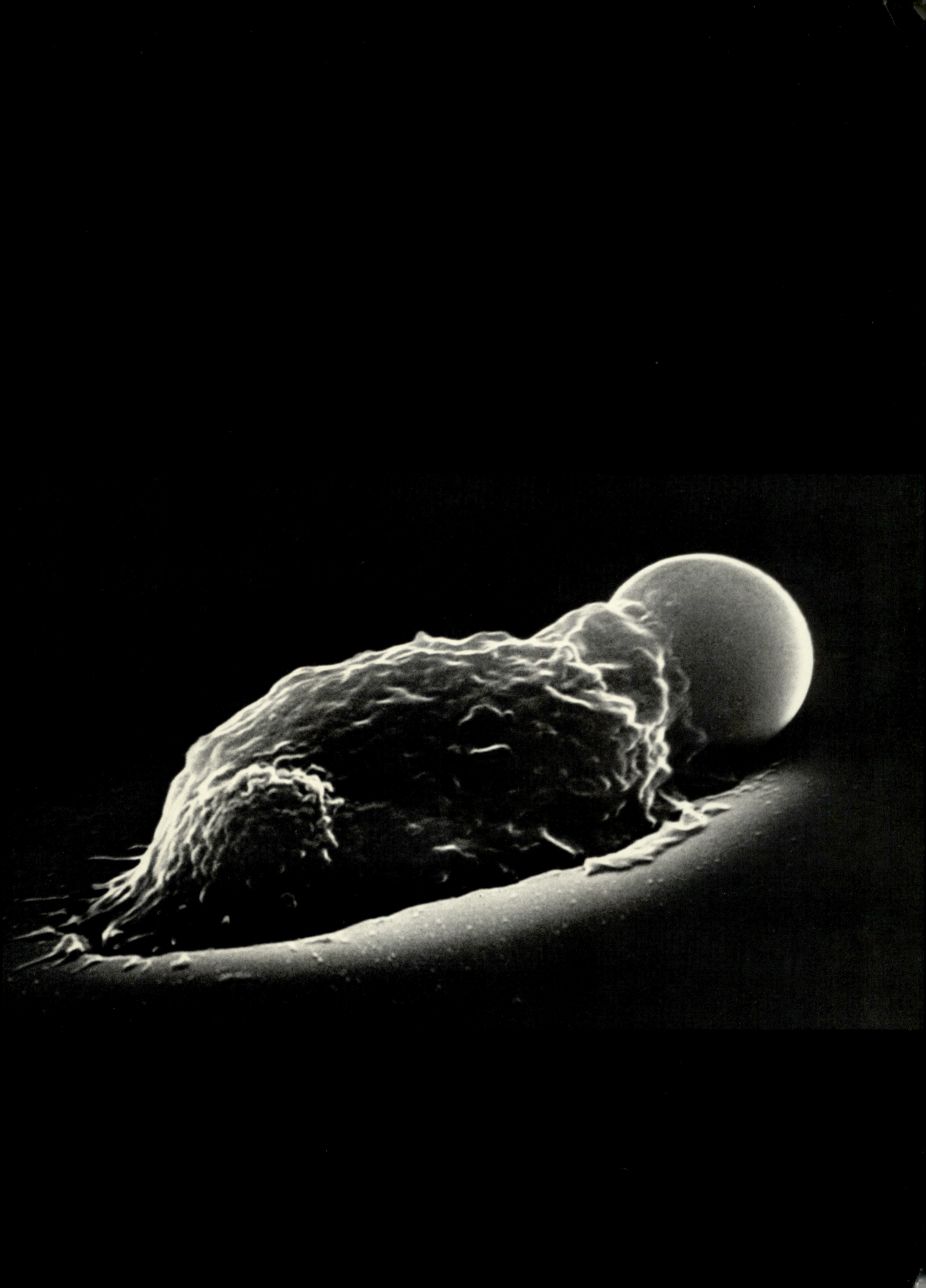

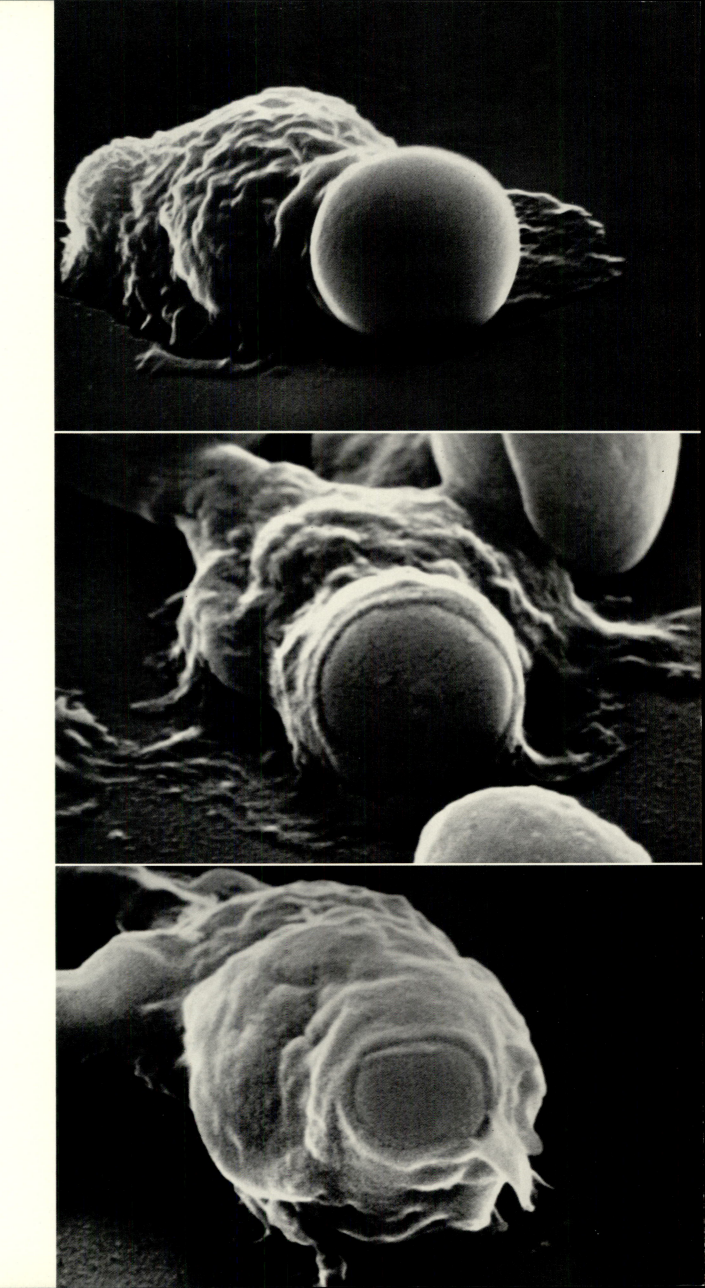

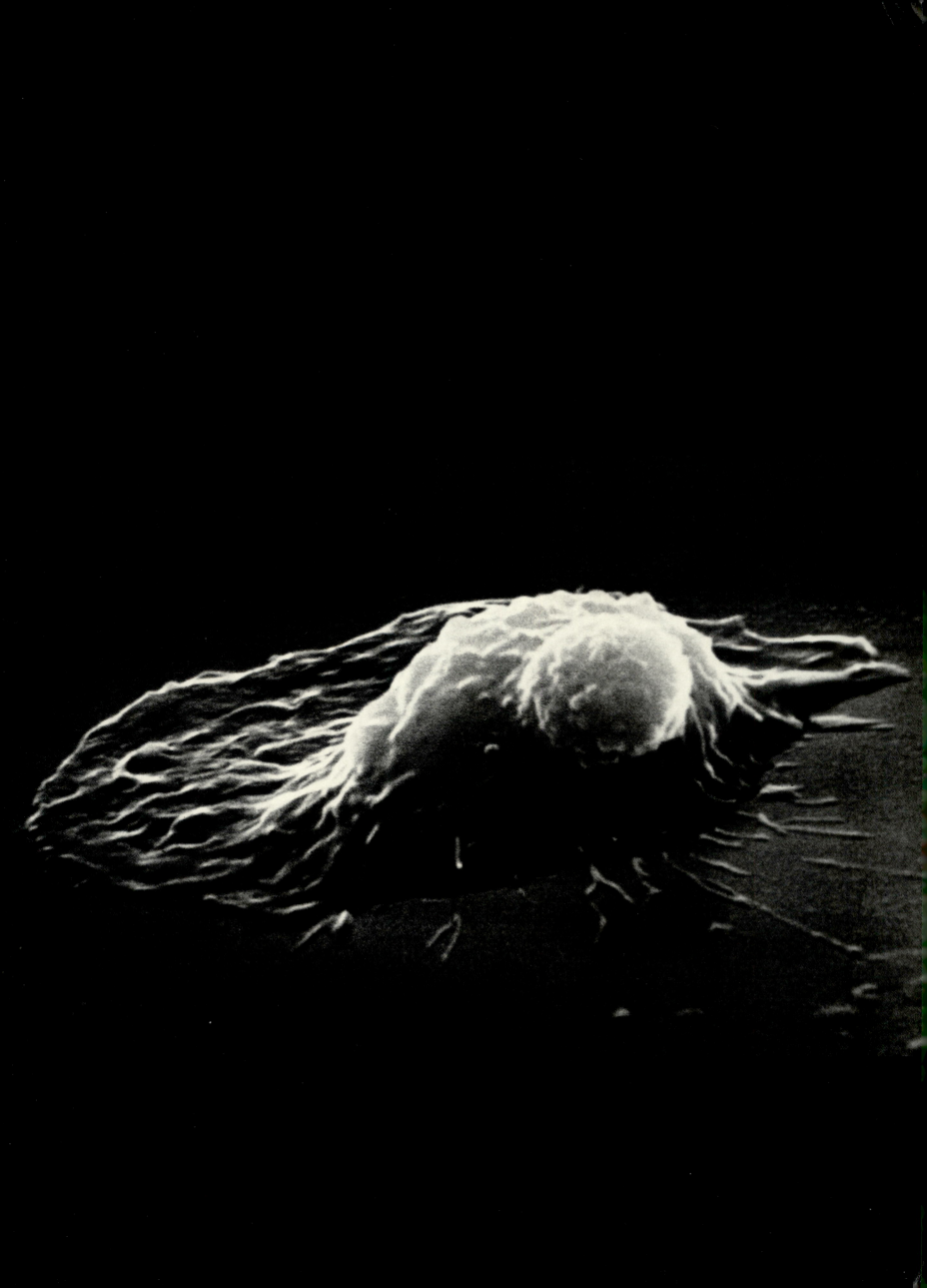

Technique and Bibliography

Technique

Blood was obtained from normal and anemic individuals. Heparin or sodium citrate was used as anticoagulant. First, a drop of fresh blood was carefully examined under the light microscope to allow thorough familiarity with the appearance of red blood cells in the living state and under different environmental conditions.

Cells were examined in whole blood, washed, oxygenized and deoxygenized, with added echinogenic or stomatogenic substances, between glass or plastic slides and coverslips and under other special conditions. Then, a drop of the suspension containing the red cells was allowed to fall into the fixative solution, the role of which is to harden and preserve the cells in the very shapes they had in their living state.

Gluteraldehyde (0.3%) and osmic acid (2%) have been used as fixatives, either singly or in combination, sometimes one after the other. Although these fixatives are considered to be the best, they do not prevent all artifacts, which one must learn to recognize. For example, under certain conditions echinocytes revert to discocytes in the process of fixation. Occasionally, freeze-drying or "critical-point technique" may be used to avoid artifacts.

After fixation it is necessary to wash the cells several times with distilled water in order to remove any protein, salt, crystals or other material that might have been deposited on the cell surface.

Next, cells must be dehydrated in preparation for desiccation, which is essential since examination by the scanning electron microscope takes place in vacuum. Dehydration is accomplished by passing the cells through increasing concentrations of alcohol followed by propylene oxide. A small drop of the cell suspension is now allowed to spread on a glass slide: desiccation will take place almost instantaneously in room air.

Before examination with the scanning electron microscope, the cells must be coated with Gold-Palladium under vacuum. The fine layer of metal makes the surface conductive. Otherwise, electric charges accumulate at certain points and render the images rapidly unrecognizable.

The images provided by the scanning electron microscope have no value unless each step of the technique of fixation, washing, dehydration and desiccation is carefully checked by parallel examination with the light microscope. If this is done, the alterations of shape due to the technique itself are negligible at the magnifications between 5,000 and 50,000 actually used.

Bibliography

Bessis, M.: *Living Blood Cells and their Ultrastructure*. New York–Heidelberg–Berlin: Springer-Verlag, 1973.

Bessis, M., Weed, R. I.: Preparation of red blood cells (RBC) for SEM. A survey of various artifacts. SEM 1972, IIT Research Institute, Chicago, part *II*, 289 (1972).

Bessis, M., Weed, R. I., Leblond, P.: *Red Cell Shape*, physiology, pathology, ultrastructure. New York–Heidelberg–Berlin: Springer-Verlag, 1973.

Brecher, G., Bessis, M.: Present status of spiculed red cells and their relationship to the discocyte-echinocyte transformation. A critical review. Blood *40*, 333 (1972).

Bull, B. S., Kuhn, I. N.: The production of schistocytes by fibrin strands. (A scanning electron microscope study.) Blood *35*, 104 (1970).

Deuticke, B.: Transformation and restoration of biconcave shape of human erythrocytes induced by amphilic agents and changes of ionic environment. Biochim. biophys. Acta (Amst.) *163*, 494 (1968).

Jensen, W. N.: Fragmentation and the "freakish poikilocyte". Amer.J.med.Sci. *257*, 355 (1969).

Lessin, L. S., Jensen, W. N., Klug, P.: Ultrastructure of the normal and hemoglobinopathic red blood cell membrane. Freeze-etching and stereoscan electron microscopic studies. Arch.int.Med. *129*, 306 (1972).

Ponder, E.: *Hemolysis and related phenomena*. New York: Grune and Stratton, 1948, reissued edition, 1971.

Ponder, E.: *Red cell structure and its breakdown*. Wien: Springer-Verlag, 1955.

Weed, R. I., LaCelle, P. L. Merrill, E. W.: Metabolic dependence of red cell deformability. J.clin.Invest. *48*, 795 (1969).

Acknowledgements

This atlas was compiled at the

Institut de Pathologie Cellulaire
INSERM unité 48
Hôpital de Bicêtre, Paris, France

with the assistance of
Anne de Boisfleury, Genevieve Prenant
and
Nicole Mercier, Pierre Mandon, Joelle Maigné

Jacques-Louis Binet and Robert I. Weed
took part in the selection of the illustrations

Marylin Nahas and Humbert Smith
helped with the English translation

George Brecher
friend and critic, edited the manuscript and improved it